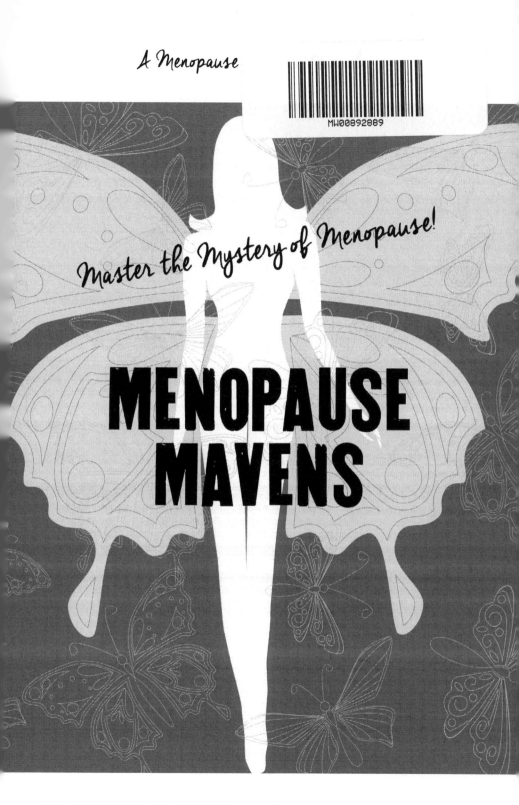

A Menopause

Master the Mystery of Menopause!

MENOPAUSE MAVENS

CO-AUTHORED BY JANE ASHLEY & VANESSA CHAMBERLIN

WITH CONTRIBUTIONS FROM 25 MARVELOUS MAVENS

FLOWER OF LIFE
PRESS.

Voices of Transformation

Published by:
Flower of Life Press™
Lyme, CT

www.floweroflifepress.com
Jane Ashley, *Publisher*

Copyright © 2015 Flower of Life Press™

ISBN 978-1503009165

Contents

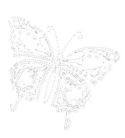

Dedication

To all of the daughters who ever were, or ever will be.

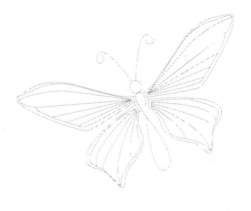

*100% of the profits of Amazon sales of this book
are being donated to the National Coalition
Against Domestic Violence (NCADV),
www.ncadv.org*

*Our donations will be used to support NCADV'S
vision to create a culture where domestic violence is
not tolerated, and where society empowers victims and
survivors, and holds abusers accountable.*

*NCADV is the catalyst for changing society to have
zero tolerance for domestic violence. They do this by
effecting public policy, increasing understanding of
the impact of domestic violence, and providing
programs and education that drive that change.*

Thank you for your support in this mission.

Introduction

BY JANE ASHLEY, *PUBLISHER*

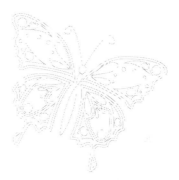

Even on the day my friend and client Vanessa said, "Get ready for this—I am in menopause!" and I said, "Holy sh*t—me too!" we had no idea how many Sisters would come forward to say, "Help me figure this out please!"

Seriously… how can a generation of woman be so confused about something that we all know is going to happen—yet are not prepared for?

Last year, I attended the Woman's Wellness Conference in San Diego. Menopause was a lead topic, with David Wolfe leading the way with amazing nutritional information, and Sara Gottfried and Lissa Rankin offering their views and solutions. Even with this wealth of information and expert advice, big questions still were arriving along with the super hot flashes and the "Hey, do you have a bath towel I can dry off with?"

So Menopause Mavens came to life, from a pure desire to ask the right questions, find answers, and offer a forum for all of us to share the good, the bad… and the parts that really suck!

This book contains a collection of essays that really hit the mark. Each woman shares her own personal journey on this path of transformation called Menopause and offers insights, tips, empathy, and her creative essence in an effort to light the path for other women.

It is more than a just a compilation of stories—it is the center of the energy that we all are bringing to this quest, the search to understand the cycle we are in, and how to discern and use all of the tools available to ease this transition of womanhood.

It's time to find new ways to communicate with each other in sisterhood so that we may find solutions and support as we travel together on the planet.

I am so honored to share these essays with you in order to ease the changes we must all go through, and embrace our lives as sacred, vital, and full of potential.

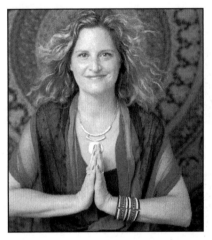

Jane Ashley is the Publisher of Flower of Life Press and is the creator of this collaborative book project, "Menopause Mavens: Master the Mystery of Menopause." Jane holds a master's degree in Transpersonal Counseling Psychology/ Art Therapy from Naropa University, and completed Nutrition training at the Institute for Integrative Nutrition. She was a featured guest speaker at IIN's 2012 fall conference at Lincoln Center in New York City.

Prior to starting Flower of Life Press, Jane was Creative Director for the Globe Pequot Press, a book publisher based in Guilford, Connecticut, where she managed a team of eight award-winning designers and was the creative leader for the company in the US and the UK. While there she art directed the New York Times bestselling books Crazy Sexy Cancer Tips *and* Crazy Sexy Survivor *by Kris Carr.*

Some of Jane's former clients include TimeWarner, Inc., the McGraw-Hill Companies, Amex, FedEx, and IBM as well as many successful coaches and wellness professionals. Jane knows the hurdles in launching a business, finding time for self-care, being with family, and the importance of collaboration in this new economy.

Her passion is to help women elevate their consciousness, lives, and businesses—by distilling their essence and creating a deep emotional connection through their message—to a place they never dreamed possible, while breaking through perceived barriers to find joy and purpose in their lives.

Learn more: www.floweroflifepress.com
Email: Jane@FlowerofLifePress.com

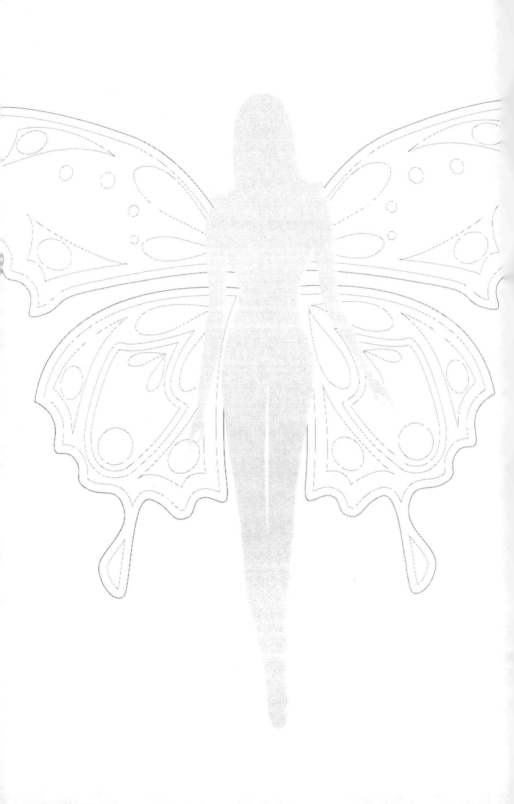

Fire-Driven

VANESSA CHAMBERLIN

Eight years ago, a knock on the door changed the course of my life. A woman with a clipboard—a coroner—told me that my husband had taken his own life.

Instantly, the only foundation I had really ever known had just been pulled from beneath me.

Two weeks later I found myself balled up on my bedroom floor with a choice to make. Would I remain a victim of this tragic circumstance, or would I dig deep within me to find the good in all that still remained? As emotionally battered as I was, I chose to stand tall and to be grateful for the amazing life we had shared together. He had been an awesome dad, stepping up to raise my older daughter Brittany as his own. And together we had two more beautiful daughters, Bianca and Bella, who needed me.

I had no idea what my new path would be, but I knew that something would show up to guide and lead me in the right direction.

Not long after my husband's death, a girlfriend called to tell me about a company and product centered on plant-based nutrition. She was over the moon about it, and soon I was too. I fell in love with the idea that nutrition really could help heal our bodies. I had found a path that made my heart sing.

I began hosting wellness events and sharing newfound knowledge of nutrition any chance I got. It was clear that by making some simple dietary changes to my family's diet—like eliminating artificial sweeteners and chemicals—positive changes were taking place, such as in my daughters' behavior and in their overall well-being.

In time, I found love again as well. And my new man—soon to be my husband—was on board with my passion for nutrition.

Three separate people told me about the same nutrition-related book, and I guess the third time was the charm. *The China Study* by Dr. Colin T. Campbell tells the story of the largest nutritional study ever performed. The findings make one very compelling point—that most major diseases are fueled by the amount of animal protein a person ingests. In a nutshell, *The China Study* says that the more plant-based foods we consume the healthier we are. I distinctly remember the conversation I had with my husband the moment I finished the book. "Hey honey, we are going plant-based/no oil tomorrow." And what he said would be the envy of many of my girlfriends: "Okay, I'm in." I can be very persuasive when I am on purpose and in my passion!

The moment I changed my diet, everything got better. When I say everything got better, I truly mean *everything*. My energy was suddenly through the roof. My passion for life, my relationships, my desire to live an even more fulfilling life, my skin, my hair, and my nails were all looking better than ever. Life was suddenly in full color. My outlook on life had never been brighter or more focused. I told my husband that I was on fire and wanted everyone to have what I had.

I devoured books on health and wellness, and I began collecting health and wellness teaching certifications like one might collect designer shoes. I attended as many conferences, lectures, and nutrition classes as I could, and I added yoga and meditation to my healthy toolbox. My goals weren't only health for myself and my family but to become an informed and inspired teacher.

I really was a girl on fire so it only seemed natural that I would create a business around the fire that burned so brightly inside of me. I dubbed my plant-based way of eating as Plantfire. The way I saw it, eating plants had given me the energy and passion to step up in my own life. Plant-based living ignited my fire within. I created an incredible community around the plant-based lifestyle. As a lifestyle coach, I taught people to love themselves from the inside out. I was shooting videos, speaking, and becoming the mom I never thought I could be. Driven to share what I've learned about nutrition and health, I published my first book, *The Fire-Driven Life: How to Ignite the Fire to Self-Worth, Health, and Happiness with a Plant-Based Diet*. I felt incredible, perhaps even unstoppable.

But something was gradually changing. It was a slow shift, but it was as if the passion I had come to know was slowly being deflated like a balloon with a leak. My energy dipped, and I was noticeably more tired. A fragility began to surface. I couldn't get enough sleep. I felt overwhelmed. My memory began to fade; simple things like someone's name or a song title would completely escape me. My workouts had always been something I enjoyed, and now I was beginning to dread them. I also noticed a change in my desire to keep building my business—something that had given me such energy in the past. I tried my best to guard my feelings, especially since I had been so vocal about how my diet and lifestyle had dramatically changed my life for good.

Self-doubt found its way in. Where I once felt a vivacious confidence when I would step into a room full of people I now found myself feeling more like a shrinking violet. I began to question my life's purpose. I had fallen into what can only be described as quiet despair. I was drifting away from the life I had built for myself, and I didn't know how to stop it. I thought that I had found the answer to the healthiest most energetic life with a plant-based diet and lifestyle. In my mind, I was doing everything right to be healthy and happy. I worked out daily, meditated twice a day, ate a beautiful plant-based diet, had a loving partner and great friends... Why did I feel like I was falling apart?

As months passed, suicidal thoughts crept in. This scared me to the point that I finally opened up to my husband about all that I hadn't articulated until that point—that my internal fire was becoming more and more dim. I was overcome by exhaustion. Even after eight hours of sleep I would wake up with the feeling that the sky was falling in. I had all but stopped teaching classes. Who was *I* to inspire others? As my own health began to falter, I began to feel like a fraud.

At forty-three years old with a life most dream of living, I was falling apart and I had no clue what to do about it. Even my periods were becoming erratic. For the first time in my life other than when I was pregnant, I had missed my period. The following month I would just have one spot and then nothing.

I decided that maybe I just needed to slow down; I had been so excited about what I was creating in life that maybe it was the universe's way of saying slow down. I didn't like that, but I listened and decided to take heed and spend more time in my own personal self-care to help give my body a rest from my self-induced overly scheduled life. But when I slowed down, the symptoms didn't disappear; instead they seemed to be screaming even louder.

By November I began to have difficulty sleeping. After practically falling into bed from exhaustion, I would wake in the middle of the night in a cold sweat. I would eventually go back to sleep but with the back of my neck drenching wet. In the beginning it started out as one or two episodes a night, but then it began to escalate. Something had to give.

That weekend I was attending a charity gala event and I suddenly felt a warm wave of heat come over me. I turned to my girlfriend and told her what I had just experienced. "Vanessa," she said, "you just had a hot flash." I described what I had been going through the last few weeks, and she said, "I think you're starting perimenopause."

"But I just turned forty-four," I said. "I'm way too young for that!"

But I wasn't. And I had missed all the symptoms. My girlfriend, who was a decade older, told me what menopause had looked like for her and that all of my signs and symptoms pointed to menopause. She gave me the name and number of a hormone specialist physician who she highly recommended. I told her about my reservations with western medicine and medication. My friend said the referral was for a doctor who works with bio-identical—not synthetic—hormones. Unconvinced, I politely tucked the doctor's number into my evening bag.

The following couple of weeks I had as many as ten night sweats a night, and, with so little sleep, I began to feel like I was going crazy. I was having what I could only describe as hot flashes throughout the day without any sort of rhyme or reason. My temper was rising faster than I could manage it. Everyday little things were beginning to really get under my skin. My patience for life itself was at an all-time low. One of the final straws that broke the camel's back happened one evening as I was preparing for dinner with my youngest daughter Bella. She made some kind of rude remark, and I had what can only be described as one of those slow-motion movie moments when I completely and instantly felt out of control of my mind and body. I threw a handful of silverware on the Travertine tile floor as hard as I could. I saw the look of shock on Bella's face, and I calmly walked myself straight back to my bedroom and locked the door behind me. I had officially lost control; I had just experienced rage. And that's what it took for me to get out that referral and make an appointment.

After having lab work done, I dragged myself to my 8 a.m. appointment with Dr. Valerie Davidson with a desperate hope in my heart that I would find some answers and relief for what I had been experiencing.

Dr. Davidson was unlike any other doctor I've met. She wanted to know not only my symptoms but about me, my life, and my beliefs. I told her that after finally realizing that I was in some sort of menopausal state I had more than likely been experiencing a hormonal decline since my early thirties. I had difficulty getting pregnant and had ended up having two in vitro fertilization pregnancies with my two younger daughters. By the time I came to see Dr. Davidson, my symptoms included itchy skin, hot flashes, night sweats, emotional outbursts, depression, decreased sex drive, and lack of focus. With every symptom that I shared, I knew I was being heard.

Dr. Davidson listened as I shared my concerns about western medicine and pharmaceuticals. She explained the difference between synthetic hormones and bio-identical ones. While both forms of hormones might stop an immediate symptom, bio-identical hormones had been proven to actually rebuild our hormones and the resulting health that comes from healthy hormone levels.

Finally, we reviewed my bloodwork. Though it was clear that my diet and lifestyle had played a critical role in the overall excellent results from my bloodwork, almost all of my hormone levels were at postmenopausal levels. Dr. Davidson assured me that having only missed two periods I was definitely not postmenopausal yet. But now every symptom I was feeling made total sense! My body was so drastically depleted of extremely important hormones that my body had no choice but to revolt against me in every way possible.

Typically, one of the first recommendations as a patient deals with menopause is that they cut back on or eliminate dairy, caffeine, and processed junk foods from their diets. This, along with meditation and yoga, were also great ways to help ease symptoms associated with menopause. Fortunately, I was already doing all of the things that were in my control. But it was clear that I was not going to eat my way, yoga my way, or meditate my way out of menopause and its natural effects on hormone levels. Dr. Davidson explained that sometimes when our body gets certain hormone levels back to a healthier range, the hormones can be triggered to jumpstart themselves. With that in mind, we decided to start with a conservative approach, even though all my hormone levels were extremely low. I would begin using estrogen cream twice a day, a progesterone pill at bedtime, and a thyroid pill first thing in the morning. After three months we would do more lab work to see how things were progressing. I understood that it can take time to get the right dosage. But at this point I was willing to try almost anything.

The body's natural state with healthy levels of hormones relies on our menstrual cycles to shed the uterus lining that builds up with hormones every month. Dr. Davidson thought that I could get my own menstrual cycle to return, and this felt like a gift. I had always had easy noneventful periods, especially after going plant-based. So, when my period suddenly stopped showing up, it felt oddly like I had lost a friend; she just vanished without any warning.

As I drove home, I began to cry in relief. I wasn't going crazy; I was going through menopause. I was still hot and irritable, but at least I was a little more at peace with my situation. I truly was a girl on fire! I knew from this point forward the relationship that I would have with my hormonal doctor would be one that would require a true partnership.

The next day felt like Christmas morning as my hormone prescription arrived from the pharmacy. Within just a few days, my symptoms were disappearing. By day 4, I was sleeping restfully. My night sweats were gone and only a handful of hot flashes were felt until they too stopped showing up. Within a couple of weeks I had a noticeable and positive change in my memory. And the best part? The sun seemed to shine bright again. The depressive fog that had creeped in and all but taken over my mind and body was finally lifting. My naturally high energy level returned, as well as my passion and drive.

I was back on the healthy happy train, and I wanted the world to know about it! I began asking everyone I knew if they were going through menopause. No one was off limits, as I figured that every man, woman, and child would in some way have experienced menopause and its wrath in some form or another. I met women who were having symptoms without realizing they were in menopause. And I met women who had already gone through the change and had done so alone and overwhelmed by the symptoms. There was no one to help usher them lovingly through the process. Every time the subject came up, it felt like I had just created the "Me too club!" The female bonding that has happened over the topic of menopause has been incredible. It has actually been part of the catalyst for me in creating more self-care through my female relationships.

I continued to feel better, and my latest bloodwork showed a marked improvement. We added a small dose of testosterone cream my last doctor visit and now I am noticing that my libido is beginning to sing again.

The road back hasn't been perfect. Sometimes I feel like getting my hormones in balance is akin to a science project. I've had breakthrough bleeding. And hormone replacement is a much-debated hot topic. It's also a very personal decision. For me, the quality of life was so diminished that riding the natural wave without any hormonal help wasn't the answer for me.

Menopause has many different faces. Some women I've spoken to describe menopause as a non-event. And for others it's been just short of a nightmare.

Too few people talk about menopause. Once I had a name for what I was going through, I wanted my husband and daughters to understand. With my girls, I am conscious of breaking the cycle of secrecy and shame around menopause. There is no stigma, and it's not an "old lady" thing. I am young vibrant and sexy *and* I am going through menopause.

One of the more important lessons I've learned is that self-care was now and forevermore be a non-negotiable to my health and happiness. My body and soul were crying out for tending loving care through friendships, healthy plant-based foods, massage, and plenty of inner reflection.

As excited as I am for what my future holds, there's still some sadness when I reflect on a chapter of my life coming to a close. I face the reality that my life is passing by so quickly.

But all I can do is live it.

And I'll leave you with a moment that made me giggle.

Bella overheard me talking with her father about perimenopause.

"Uncle Perry has menopause?" she said, excitedly. "Does Aunt Casie know?"

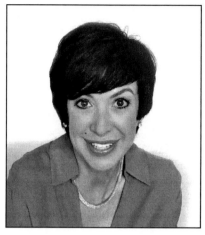

Vanessa Chamberlin grew up in a typical American family, eating the meat, starch, and sugar-laden fare that was standard everywhere. She knew it didn't feel right and that she didn't want to grow up to be overweight and sick like most of the adults around her.

Fast forward to 2008. Vanessa had tried low-fat, low-carb, Fen-Phen, grapefruit, cabbage soup, and every other fad that grabbed the public attention. Her ah-hah moment came when she read The China Study, *T. Colin Campbell's ground-breaking work that de-bunked almost every western food tradition. The next day, literally, Vanessa changed her diet for herself and her family. In an instant she said goodbye to unhealthy food and hello to a plant-based diet that she calls PlantFire!*

To better understand her newfound appreciation of healthy whole foods, Vanessa widened her studies to include nutrition and coaching certifications from the Institute of Integrative Nutrition, The Institute for the Psychology of Eating, Cornell University, SUNY Purchase, and the Wellness Forum, where she is certified as a Lifestyle Medicine Practitioner. She is accredited through the American Association of Drugless Practitioners (AADP), is a member of the national charity league, and is a board member of both Create A Change Now and The Miss Nevada Scholarship Organization. Throw in her certification from the Yoga Alliance, and Vanessa is uniquely qualified to bring the Fire-Driven lifestyle to a public sorely in need of powerful, meaningful change.

Today, Vanessa is dedicated to bringing the message of wellness to as many people as possible, and her Fire-Driven lifestyle includes a TV series, several books, and various events centered on the PlantFire cooking and cuisine she loves. She is a sought-after speaker and coach and also owns Vasari, a luxury clothing and shoe boutique in Las Vegas.

*Learn more: **www.VanessaChamberlin.com***

2

Reclaiming Our Feminine Energy

MUNEEZA AHMED

I am a young goddess in my thirties, and I never imagined that I would be writing a chapter in a book about menopause. But as a good friend of mine said, "You work with women in menopause and perimenopause all the time, so I guess it does make sense."

Menopause is this huge dreaded change for most women. In fact for most women, all of their so-called changes—during puberty, menstruation, labor and birth, and especially menopause—are dreaded. Girls changing into women can be a scary and confusing time. Women typically do not welcome their monthly cycles with joy—rather, it is another dreaded time for them. And we certainly don't as a culture welcome labor and birth. Birth is usually a very unwelcome and horrific experience for women. I should know—I teach natural birthing classes and I listen to hundreds of women's fears around birth. So then why would menopause be any different?

Although I want to talk about menopause, I *really* want to address what is it that we resist about women's bodies and our emotional and spiritual makeup.

Somewhere in history our culture turned into a patriarchal one. A long time ago especially in the times of Lemeuria (ancient land on earth) we used to live in a matriarchal culture. This slowly shifted into a more patriarchal culture and one that imposed the idea of separation and the subjugation of women or the feminine arche-type, including qualities like magnetic attraction and manifestation, intuition, honoring of our emotional unpredictability, not moving in a straight line, and surrender.

We are created in our feminine to balance with the masculine. This is evident in the basis of creation of the flower of life (the feminine, circular form), in which is embedded the metatron's cube, the geometric, linear, masculine form. The masculine and feminine were always intended to balance and live in complete harmony and resonance, but clearly we have moved far away from that in our world today.

The problem with the patriarchal culture today is the loss of recognition of the feminine balance. And its not just men who have lost this recognition, it is women also. The reason that our hormonal cycles are so out of balance is that we are living far too much from our masculine energies and not enough from the feminine.

Every human being, male or female, has masculine and feminine energies. For example, just as a woman has the capability to be soft and vulnerable (a feminine strength) she also has the capability to be directional and goal focused (a masculine energy). It is similar for men. Men are hunters or providers by nature (think of what sperm do, a masculine energy), yet they have the capability to be in touch with their emotions (a more feminine quality). The problem today is that men are out of balance with their feminine (heart energy) and women are also out of touch with their feminine energy. Women are working more and more in corporate situations alongside men, dressing like men, talking like men and not acknowledging any of their feminine qualities or needs. It is not just true for women in the corporate world; women all over have adopted a masculine stance and are really disconnected from their feminine selves. This is evidenced in all the hormonal problems we witness in our bodies today.

There is nothing WRONG with women's bodies, they are just not functioning with the right fuel. Imagine if you put in diesel fuel into a car engine that needs only unleaded fuel, the result is not going to be a great functioning car. Likewise, what women really need to ease all of the physical burdens of their body cycles is to connect with their feminine energy.

My deepest belief is that there is no need to experience the difficult physical symptoms of menopause—the vaginal dryness, weight gain, the loss of libido, loss of skin elasticity, the mood swings, or the hot flashes.

I know that the myth of having painful births has been busted by many women including myself (I have had three pain-free births, with no medical interventions—in fact, a couple of my births were orgasmic!). This tells me deep in my feminine knowing that menopause does not need to be experienced by women in a difficult way either. Women in touch with their feminine essence, their sensuality, and their pleasure can experience menopause gracefully and beautifully. In fact the feminine design calls for pleasure through all experiences. And by pleasure I don't mean orgasm, but I do mean the energy of feeling that good—the energy of feeling orgasmic.

I am a medical intuitive. So in that regard I also feel it's essential for me to share that the basis for all great health is to eat right and to include supplements that really serve women's health. I will outline a few of them here.

Many of the issues around menopause surround the endocrine system, and if you haven't reached menopause yet, it's a great idea to focus on keeping your endocrine system healthy. After all, the hormones of our body are the gateway between our physical and spiritual selves. Some great foods and supplements to include before and during the change are as follows. (Some of this information was taught to me by Anthony William, Medical Medium, www. medicalmedium.com/book):

- Barley grass juice powder (for alkalinity)
- Bio-identical progesterone (organic excellence brand by John Lee)
- Sweet potatoes
- Avocados
- Coconuts (water, butter, fruit and oil)
- Magnesium (ancient minerals bath flakes and lotion)
- Shatavari (powdered herb—from organic india or longevity-warehouse.com)
- Dong Quai (Angelica root)
- Detoxadine (iodine from Global Healing Center)
- Winter squashes
- Berries of all kinds, especially wild blueberries

It is really important to include foods in this topic because we are discussing hormones, which are physical energies in our bodies. And given that we live in a physical body, we need to address foods and supplements that affect our physical bodies. When we can support our physical bodies, we support the gateway to our spiritual being.

During hormonal changes in the body, women can sometimes struggle with fatigue and weight gain, not because of the change itself but because the hormonal change may trigger underlying viruses in the liver and the thyroid. In fact, according to Anthony William, Medical Medium,® the majority of thyroid disease is triggered by an underlying virus in the thyroid gland. This is one of the main reasons to include iodine in the diet and barley grass juice powder, because these two supplements greatly support the thyroid gland and, if taken prior to a hormonal change, can mitigate the effects of any underlying virus. I regularly consult with women in my practice on these topics and help them move through changes as gracefully and easily as possible.

One of the major reasons women struggle through hormonal changes is because they are disconnected from the main marker of their health, which is their libido. Having a low libido is a sure sign of other hormonal systems in the body being off. Here is where I want to talk more about women and their connection to their pleasure.

We are so in the mode of giving and living from depletion that we have come to accept as normal this feeling of disconnection and exhaustion. While exhaustion can be another symptom of an underlying virus trigger like I mentioned earlier, the disconnection from pleasure and feeling good is because of the hormonal imbalance. We have become disconnected from our intuition, from knowing what makes us feel good, and from taking right action. Turning this around can seem overwhelming, so committing everyday for just 10 or 15 minutes to doing something in your pleasure is a good starting point.

Womankind is capable of immense pleasure. The key to living from our feminine space—which I have seen in my practice do wonders for the female hormonal system—is to connect with our pleasure in simple every life tasks, as well as in bed. Helping women reconnect with their pleasure has enabled them to get their period back and in many cases recover their libido as well.

Sexually, women have the ability to experience three main types of orgasm. The most common one is the clitoral orgasm. The next deepest is the G-spot orgasm and is achieved by stimulating the G-spot about 1 to 2 inches inside the vagina. The deepest orgasm is the cervical orgasm, which is achieved by stimulating the cervix, and the experience of this is often described as akin to transcendental meditation. Experiencing the deeper orgasms opens women up to their more feminine energies. They become magnetic and aroused as they "wake" up to life.

Having a practice of regularly engaging orgasmic energy, which is all at once sexual, creative (used to create life), and spiritual (brings forth new life), can bring a woman to experience more pleasure in other areas of her life.

As we learn to love our bodies, engage our pleasure, support ourselves with the right foods and supplements, and live from the feminine, we can imagine the possibility of *enjoying* menopause. The understanding that there can be viral issues that are completely reversible given the correct protocols can stop us from shaming our bodies and using crazy diets to shed weight and bring more sanity to this very important turning point in a woman's life. This time that is considered as the end of her fertility and can make women really sad can in fact be the beginning of so much more—an embodiment of the crone and the wise woman archetypes. A woman doesn't have to lose any of herself as she enters menopause.

If women can have pain-free and even orgasmic childbirth, we can certainly have orgasmic and pleasurable menopause.

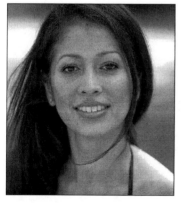

Muneeza Ahmed is a true global citizen, born in Pakistan, raised in Dubai, educated in London, and for the last 10 years has been building her business in Connecticut.

Her journey to her own health and vital energy began when lifelong allergies and asthma reached crisis stage—the unfamiliar climate and toxicity sending Muneeza to the emergency room eight times in her first year in the US. Traditional medicine had failed—the drugs didn't work—and the path of the healer began.

Muneeza is a medical intuitive, and her skills were honed as she explored alternate therapies, studied nutrition, and gained insight into energy healing—and the power of science and Spirit to create transformation. As her own health improved, her desire to share her knowledge and help others led her to a thriving practice, encompassing Intuitive Medicine, Energy Healing featuring the Body and Emotion Code, Personal Coaching and Sacred Birthing programs. Learn more: www.muneezaahmed.com.

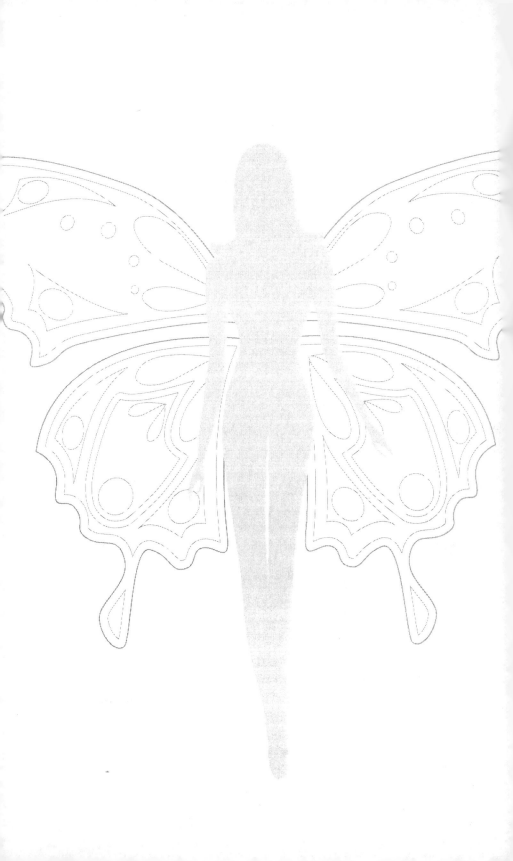

3

From the Brink and Back

MINDI ANDERSON

It all began with two aggressive rounds of in-vitro fertilization (IVF) with the hope that my husband and I would raise a child together. How naïve! Both rounds were failures. I don't know how women can go through this process five or even ten times! God bless them all.

After the IVF in late 2005 and mid-2006, and actually within a few months of the last round, life was a shit-storm. I can't describe it any other way. I had no idea what I would be in for after trying so hard to become a mother. I walked away from it, not wanting to do it again. I was done. I was broken. I had to collect myself and find my sanity, which was on the brink.

I was thirty-six and still struggling with the question: kids or no kids? Am I less than, because I didn't give birth? Does my life have less meaning without being a parent? Does this define me? And is this definition positive? I was so tired—beyond tired—*exhausted* from hearing from people say "it's okay" that I "didn't have kids" and then make suggestions as to how I might try again. That is the most degrading and patronizing thing a human could ever say to another. Did I need approval and validation from friends, family, and strangers? I was shocked and blown away by things people say about mothering and parenting in general, like there is nothing else to do while we are here on earth, or how the most important thing is to leave a legacy. It was nauseating. I have to be honest. You just do not know what this feels like until you experience it for yourself. And, honestly, I would never wish that on anyone.

A couple of months following the final round of IVF, I began to have panic episodes: nausea, the feeling of possibly fainting, head spinning, and a sense of doom washing over me from head to toe. *What was this?* I had never experienced this feeling. And it was so ironic—I didn't know at the time—that it was just out of the blue that I was now hypoglycemic. Really? Now I have blood sugar problems? I just crumbled. *One* more thing that was chipping me away to nothingness. I had no idea what was happening.

I asked myself, was this the result of all of these drugs that were injected into my body? Was this a sickness? Was I dying? Imagine yourself already stricken with panic, and now you think any little abnormality going in with your body is a terminal illness. I was a zombie. The physical and emotional aftermath was terrible. But I laugh even as I write this. I laugh now, because I look back at where I was and now where I am and I am so grateful to be here sharing this story with you.

As the months passed into years, I was slowly declining in my work teaching yoga and holistic health. My enthusiasm waned. Who was I to offer advice to others? I experienced more panic episodes, more body issues, weight gain, lethargy, and depression. My doctor at the time told me that anti-depressants and anti-anxiety medicines would be a good place to start to help with these episodes and help me to relax.

Really?, I thought, *I teach deep breathing and meditation, and I take Xanax?*

But I did.

It was such a desperate space in my life that I felt I had no other choice. You cannot see or think clearly when you feel as miserable as this felt. So I just took the two prescriptions I was given, and they did help—for a while.

Between 2008 and 2010, I was fat. Seriously, fat. Puffed up and pissed at the world. With my body on a downward spiral, I tried going gluten free, sugar free, carb free, caffeine free, dairy free, alcohol free. I went vegan and got fatter and felt even worse, I went Paleo and was beginning to look like a chicken, and finally I just had it.

The doctor who had medicated me told me that around my age (thirty-nine!) I could expect to begin to feel the effects of aging. So basically I was being put out to pasture. It's over, once you are forty, just turn yourself in and wear a Moo-Moo for the rest of your days.

My BAD-itude was projecting even more, and my client base was dwindling, my desire to even work nearly dissipated. Both in my energy and my physical appearance, I was a mess, and not a *hot* mess. No wonder people weren't queuing up to work with me. I could barely help even *myself*. I felt un-sexy, tired, overwhelmed, jealous, insecure, hungry, angry, obsessed, tortured, sad, happy, bloated, old, worn down like an old tire. I mean, it felt like my warranty had expired and there weren't any parts available for my model.

I couldn't accept it. So I fired my doctor and, then Dr. Carolyn appeared. She saved me, one hormone at a time. I was a zombie, and she helped me find my way back to a full life. She explained to me that although we all get older, how we age is not a sentence to serve.

We all get older, and aging is normal. But while conventional medicine says there's little to do about it, Dr. Carolyn disagreed. After having all of the appropriate tests and even going deeper than most doctors would do, we were both surprised that I was even functioning. The depletion of nutrients in my body and the low levels of hormones across the board were shocking. We could only assume—though we cannot be 100-percent certain—that it was due to the aggressive hormones injected during IVF. It was like my body zipped itself up and wouldn't let the drugs out. Stress was a significant factor, as my cortisol levels were through the roof and my adrenals were not just a little tired, they were depleted.

A few months after I began hormone replacement therapy, I was baffled by how good I felt. I woke up wanting to do something with my life, and I had heart and motivation and inspiration in my soul. It was not an overnight process; I still had things to deal with. But I had answers, and we cannot move forward with certain things in life—our bodies and minds—if we cannot find answers. I had hope, and I have a doctor who hugs me when I see her.

I completed my Nutrition Certification, as well as a 200-Hour Yoga Teacher Training Certification, and I am rounding the corner on my master's in psychology in behavioral health.

More importantly, I learned that I am just as important as those I care for, and I have embraced myself, flaws and all. I would *love* to have six-pack abs, but for now I will settle for the three-pack, and those are not always visible either.

I love my life, and I love that I am not ashamed that I may need medicines for certain things in life. And it's no one's business but mine if I eat steak and fries or ice cream once in a while, while enjoying my martini. It really isn't. If I have learned and embraced one thing out of all of this: I don't have to explain myself to anyone. I must be at peace with myself and go inward and take my inventory regularly.

I want you, dear reader, to find that in your heart and soul. Look at yourself every day and see how you can inspire yourself and others. You have a lot of work to do here—and a lot of fun to have. So grab it, embrace it, and treat yourself well. Find a sustainable lifestyle that works for *you*, without comparison and without judgment. There is no one blueprint for everyone.

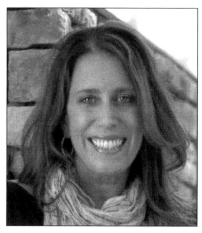

Mindi Anderson is a Behavioral Wellness Partner and a lifelong student of human psychology and how it relates to the habits we form. In 2014 she founded The Inspired Life to partner with people from all walks of life in Las Vegas, the United States, and abroad: to create individualized circles of wellness for a life of complete prosperity of mind, body, and soul. She is matriculating with a graduate degree in Behavioral Health and Psychology. Mindi enjoys playing tennis and golfing with her husband of seventeen years. A trained and certified yoga instructor, she has over 200 hours of training, coupled with certification in nutrition, making her a true partner for women seeking a balanced lifestyle.

Learn more: www.MindiAnderson.com

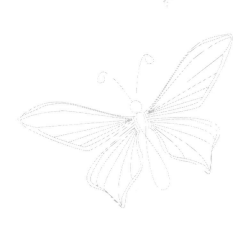

Are you there God/Goddess? It's me, Ami.

AMI BEACH

I'm deep in this dance. Sometimes it's a dance of flow, and sometimes it feels like an obstacle course. The heat is on! I am transforming and shedding my old skin. I know what's possible here—I know what's at stake, what's to lose, and what's to gain. Once again, I bow before a new altar of womanhood, and nothing short of surrender is required of me.

My personal journey into perimenopause began roughly a decade ago at age thirty-five. There were changes in my period, as it became more erratic and flowed heavier. Migraine headaches came frequently and with great intensity. Insomnia and numbness in my hands and feet became a nightly occurrence. By my late thirties, the chronic headaches and heavy menses became so crippling that, finally—after trying every herb, holistic therapy, fasting cleanse, colonic therapy and every other thing that I had mastered in own my scope of practice—I gave in to seeing a specialist who could help diagnose my situation.

After my ultrasound and examination, the doctor concluded that I had developed stage 4 endometriosis—the most severe type—and the best alternative for me was radical surgery and to place a synthetic Mirena copper intrauterine device (IUD) into my cervix to control my hormones.

As a holistic specialist, I questioned him greatly about the long-term effects of taking synthetic hormones and flat out refused to discuss a radical hysterectomy as an option. After a long debate, I agreed to try the IUD as a short-term solution to give me some relief, as he convinced me the copper IUD is "harmless, inert, and localized."

Fast forward to my fortieth birthday. By now, the IUD had been in place for about a year. Although the extreme clotting and head-aches had been reduced greatly, I had a significant list of new symp-toms that were haunting me and accumulating almost daily. Since the IUD, I had gained an unexplained twenty pounds around my midsection. I began having chronic urinary tract infections, chronic yeast infections, hives, several bouts of Epstein-Barr virus, swelling of my face, tightness in my chest, severe mental fogginess, and mood swings, just to name a few.

My moods became so drastic that I would fly off the handle with the slightest sign of stress. Some days I would lie in bed and scream aloud to the higher powers to just end my misery and pray to God/Goddess to help guide me past this dark time and show me to the light. It was in this darkest hour that I started to understand the grave importance of hormones and, in particular, estrogen dominance.

My prayers were answered when I came across a book by Dr. John R. Lee called *What Your Doctor May Not Tell You About Pre-menopause*, as well as a few books by Dr. Christiane Northrup that helped me identify with the spiritual side of the changes going on in my body. I quickly determined the synthetic hormones in the IUD were in fact making me more sick. I trusted my gut instinct and had the IUD removed. Within a week, it was out and I had a new lease on life.

The scope of my life and my private practice as a raw food life-style and detox specialist started to focus on the clear connection between our hormones and our health. I also began to connect spir-itually to the changes going on in my body. I had a new sense of liberation, freedom, and renewed hope. It became clear to me that each woman needs to trust in her own innate body's wisdom and not give her power away so quickly, like I had.

We cannot allow ourselves to be tricked by how products are misrepresented by the media, clever advertisements, or even our own doctors. In the example of the Mirena IUD, the clever advertisement slogan "Fit and Forget" is lovely but doesn't at all represent the horrific side effects that come from its use. In fact, since having it removed, I have researched more than two thousand known side effects. And although my doctor felt like he was giving me his best advice, if I had listened to him, I would likely be standing here today as a very sick woman having undergone a radical hysterectomy and possibly with something far worse like cervical cancer.

I believe with every fiber of my being that if I had continued to go down that road, my physical and mental health would have continued in a downward spiral. It was time to go within, trust myself, and allow the body to speak to me on a physical level but also, more importantly, on a deeply spiritual level.

What is the body trying to tell us during perimenopause?

Perimenopause is a time to be gentle with ourselves and reduce our expectations and commitments. Our inner self is speaking very loudly, and this is a critical time to listen. Perimenopause, like menarche, menstruation, and childbirth, is a portal into a sacred dimension of womanhood—a shift into transformation and growth.

So what is this portal into womanhood trying to show me?

Like all of the altars of womanhood, perimenopause is a deeply personal experience, both physically and mentally for all woman. However, there are common threads of insights, lessons, and wisdom that can be shared with others. Perimenopause is an exciting developmental stage that changes and transforms us at the core.

Perimenopause and all that it offers is designed to heal all the unhealed parts of you. As Dr. Christiane Northrup says, "Perimenopause is a crossroads, one road says grow, the other road says die and it feels like the end. What is required at perimenopause is a drastic change of heart, to prevent disease. It is time to fuel your life from your soul, from source energy—and do what you really want to do. Time to give up 'Perfect' and reframe 'Selfish.'"

In other words, perimenopause is a wake-up call.

Once I had the proper information about my hormones and how to balance them naturally, combined with the spiritual implications of the changes going on within my body, perimenopause became the single-most prolific, transformational time of my life. All the struggles mentally and physically that tormented me have proven to be the greatest teachers and gifts. As a detox specialist, colon hydrotherapist, raw foods chef, and longevity strategist for more than twenty years, confronting perimenopause head on was the missing link to embodying the health and vitality that I always craved. The combination of the power of a raw foods lifestyle, periodic juice fasting, natural progesterone crème (from Wild Yam and topically applied), meditation, the G-glo™ lifestyle, and total and complete unconditional acceptance of myself is what ultimately gave me back my health.

Now, I am virtually symptom free of stage 4 endometriosis, my insomnia is a thing of the past, and I feel back in my body again like I did when I was in my twenties. I am eternally grateful to have discovered the magic combination of lifestyle, natural hormones, diet, and spiritual connection that has given me my life back. In turn, I am dedicated to working with women of all ages to help empower them to also take control of the wheel of their life and claim a life of vibrant health that is their sovereign right.

At forty-four, I'm right smack dab in the middle of perimenopause and I see a place of clarity beyond the confusion. I see a space in my life where it is obvious that it's up to me and only me what magic I make in my life. I face choices and decisions about who I am in the world and in my work, how I am in my relationships, and how I experience and embrace aging.

Each visit to an altar of womanhood builds on the one before, and we see the story of our life journey as it unfolds. Our experiences at these various altars of transformation hold within them the key lessons we have come here for. As Dr. Northrup says, "Women labor as they live." This is an opportunity for personal reflection and awareness. And here, at the altar of perimenopause, I see so clearly that when my body does speak up loud and clear, it brings me directly into the present moment—the here and now. Midlife wisdom is a fusion of the mind, body, and heart. When you heal the heart, you heal the world. I realize more than ever that the work I do to heal my heart makes it easier for everyone else around me to heal their hearts, too.

So rather than focusing on struggle, fear, and any new symptoms that emerge, I bring myself directly to the here and now and the difference I can make on the world around me. I let go of the past and remain an open vessel to allow life to flow freely through me. I am eternally grateful for this rite of passage as it has allowed me to heal myself on a deeply physical level but also on an even more profoundly spiritual level than I could ever have imagined. And now, the magic unfolds daily! For this I am truly blessed and honored to share my knowledge, wisdom, and experience with womankind collectively. Namaste.

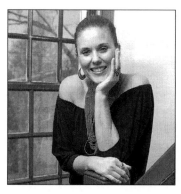

Ami Beach *has over twenty years of hands-on experience as a raw foods chef, detox specialist, holistic health coach, and colon hydrotherapist. Featured on NBC, CBS, "ABC News," First* for Women *magazine, and* Self *magazine, Ami is co-owner of G-Zen Restaurant in Branford, Connecticut, alongside her husband, celebrity master vegan chef Mark Shadle. G-Zen was named one of the Top Ten Vegan restaurants in America by* Shape *magazine. Ami successfully guided hundreds of her clients to transition into a more vibrant, raw lifestyle. Her passion is to inspire individuals to take charge of their own health by teaching powerful tools including a raw/living foods diet, juice fasting, detoxification protocols, and the importance of digestive health. Ami is also founder of the G-Glo Raw Juice Feast and Raw Radiance Diet (RRD) that have been endorsed by best-selling author Dr. Ann Louise Gittleman.*

Learn more: **www.G-Glo.com** *and* **www.g-zen.com**. *Ami tweets at mydetoxdiva.*

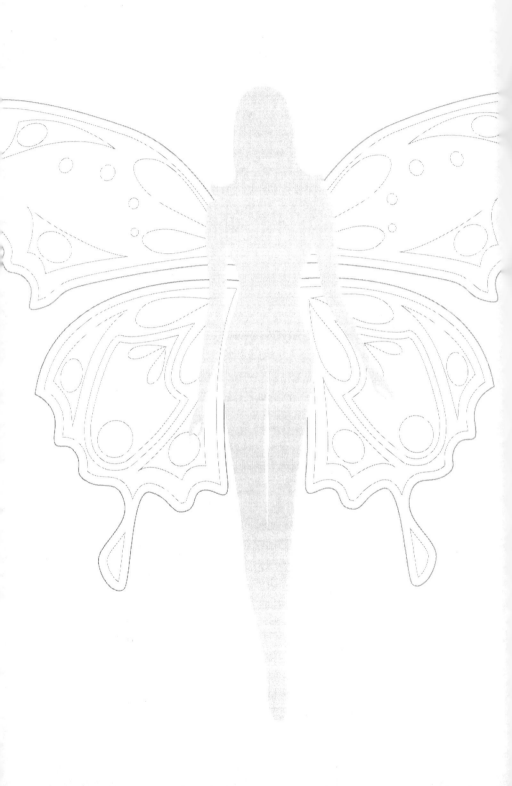

5

Truth Seeker: From Caregiver to Self-Care

JUDY BEN-ASHER

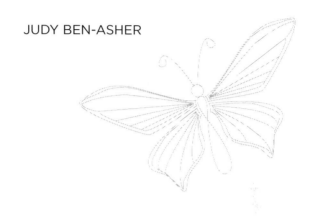

I just woke up and the first thing that is racing through my head is, "Hey I didn't wake up in a pool of sweat and my hair is still dry!" In disbelief, I run through my mind all the countless things I have tried to see which was *the* thing that worked.

I have an autoimmune disease called Hashimoto's or Hashi's. I am *not* in menopause but I have many of the same symptoms. I *thought* I was in menopause since my Hashi's went undiagnosed for basically my whole life until now. So, yep, night sweats and hot flashes that always manage to come at the worst possible times, crazy weight gain, and *holy crap* ginormous mood swings! That beautiful wet, dripping face, when I am trying to have a normal conversation with someone and it is cold outside but, yeah, I am now soaked with sweat, just dripping and trying to pretend like it's all good, no problem—this is actually happening, again!

This past year, Jane Ashley of the Menopause Mavens and I were at a David Wolfe event the Woman's Wellness Conference. For the first time, I had a hot flash buddy! It is so odd and so comforting to have someone sweating with me in a room with blasting AC, just because our bodies were like, ok, *now!* That was the first time I realized what it is we actually do go through in menopause—how big a change it really is and how we *have to* figure this out and diminish these symptoms for us all, forever!

I have been a voiceover artist for animation, as well as actor and director for the past twenty years. When my mom was diagnosed with stage IIIC ovarian cancer in 2011, I didn't know all that much about health. But, as anyone who is dealing with cancer knows, you get educated *really* quickly. Cancer is like a train you chase until it's over. My mom had lost many organs in her first surgery; they resected her colon, took out her gallbladder and omentum (the layer of the peritoneum that surrounds the abdomen and stores needed fat), and shortened her intestine. Knowing her nutrition would be a challenge, I dove into research to find solutions. I was searching for a faster way to help her heal, what to feed her, and how to get optimal nutrition for her. I knew we had to reduce her inflammation, nourish her body, and get cancer-fighting food in.

David Wolfe was the first nutrition expert and researcher I found whose work made sense to me. I read everything I could get my hands on. I wanted to learn even more so I went back to school for integrative nutrition. The more I learned about actual nutrition, the angrier I felt at all the misinformation. It is not our fault that we believe the diet industry and medical field; we were raised to. But the more I learned about cancer, who was profiting and what was going on with my own body, I felt like I *had to do something about it* and share what I was learning.

At the time, I was more than 100 pounds overweight though I worked out often and ate what I thought was very healthy. I was not a heavy child but started gaining weight in my teens and never stopped—until now at age forty-five. I had no idea why my body didn't work like everyone else's. No matter what I ate, I gained weight. I was a vegetarian for thirty-one years starting at ten years old. I was now learning that my version of a veggie diet was more like fast food vegetarian—not so good!

One of the biggest gifts I received while attending The Institute for Integrative Nutrition was learning about bio-individuality. It means that we are *not* all the same and we *should not* all be doing the same thing for our health but rather what is best for us as individuals. This concept was a *huge* revelation for me! The diet industry keeps misinforming us about all these fad diet and new products. Throughout my life, I had experienced shame in seeking new options for myself as I tried to figure it out. People in my life were getting sick of hearing about "my weight" and why I was trying everything just to feel better. More than once I was told, "Just see a doctor and take a pill! Or get your stomach stapled." I, too, was sick of talking about it all the time and didn't want to spend another day feeling like crap.

I began to dive in deeper and meet and interview people from many backgrounds in the health industry to learn how to feed my mom so that she would hopefully live—and also to heal myself. On my journey I learned some powerful lessons and gifts. My biggest lesson was that just because I want my mom to eat certain foods to help her heal, she may not choose to do so! She wanted to eat what she wanted to eat, period. I had to surrender and accept that she was in charge of her health, as she should be. My mom fought hard. Tragically, in June 2014, we lost her.

As a result of my mom's illness and my own experience with Hashimoto's, I am filming a documentary called "TruthSeeker" in an effort to help us all find our best level of health. In the film, we explore how our thoughts and belief systems set up our life and death and how to shift them forever. We dispel misinformation on nutrition, dive into hormonal balancing, thyroid, menopause, exercise, and meditation to have our best lives ever.

During this process of learning, I discovered that I *could* do something about the autoimmune disease Hashimoto's that I suffered from. I needed to start with my own belief systems and completely change my eating. I also realized that I needed to set up clearer boundaries with the people around me who were unsupportive. As my life was changing and shifting, I began to feel empowered with this new knowledge, and I am proud to be able to share it with you in the "TruthSeeker" film and related book. After losing my mom, I have an even stronger desire to *live* my best and happiest life—and share what I've learned.

I am currently following an eating plan that I created for my Hashimoto's disease that is really diminishing my menopause symptoms. It is an autoimmune diet that avoids foods that are irritants and are anti-inflammatory and alkalizing. A major lesson I am learning is that most imbalance and disease comes from inflammation in our system, so I removed grains, sugar, dairy, nightshades, nuts, seeds, caffeine, and alcohol. I will adjust this diet as I heal, but for now, I am losing about a pound a day. Some weeks the weight loss has been less but I am still consistently dropping. I sleep better than I have my whole life. I have not had any night sweats or hot flashes. The cravings that used to rule my day are gone! YAY!

After all the research I have done, I believe that an anti-inflammatory, alkalizing diet is the best way to go—for most of us. If we take the inflammation out and eat very clean and healthy foods, we will feel better and our bodies will function more optimally. I am living proof of that.

Meditation and Pilates have made a massive difference in how I feel, too. Instead of a gym membership, I bought myself a Pilates Reformer on Amazon—the best gift I have ever given myself! It has a rebounder attachment that really gets the lymph moving. My body feels great but not overly exhausted, and it is very low impact on my joints and knees. After having so much extra weight for so long, my knees are fragile to say the least.

When it comes to being a Menopause Maven, there are so many amazing ways we can get through this transition gently. As women, we are so powerful when we come together and support each other. When we pool our resources and share information, we surely will find out what is best for our own bio-individuality. How lucky are we to have such a smart and strong tribe of TruthSeekers?!

We can heal ourselves.
We can feel better.
We can get through this gracefully and with dignity, together!

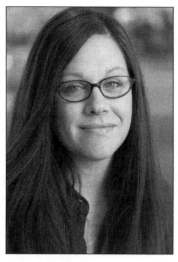

Judy Ben-Asher has worked in film as an actor, voice-over artist, director, producer, writer, and filmmaker. When her mother became ill in 2011, she attended The Institute for Integrative Nutrition, becoming a health coach. Later that year she studied with Terry Hickey and the Holistic MBA program, becoming a Transformational Coach. Judy began her journey of discovery to find out how to help save her mom from cancer. Sadly, she had barely begun to interview when her mom passed. Instead of stopping, Judy shifted—her need to understand deepened by loss as well as by her own life-threatening health imbalances. With courage and an open mind, Judy has pulled leading minds to discuss and to question, searching for keys to wellness. She is currently filming a documentary called "TruthSeeker, Shedding Layers and Shifting Forward."

Learn more: *www.TruthSeekerFilms.com*

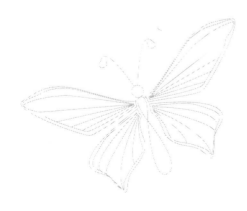

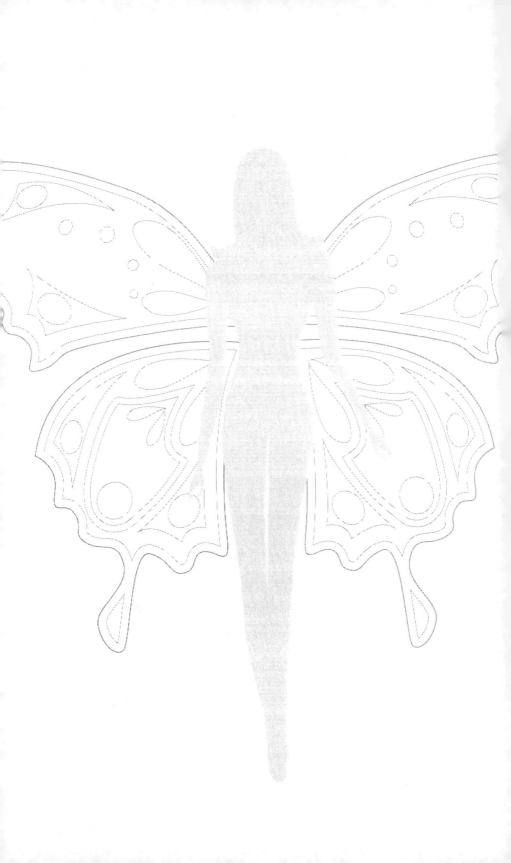

6

The change: Keeping It Lowercase

GRACE CADDELL

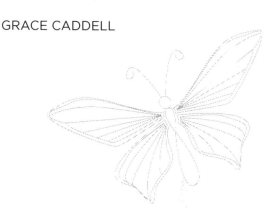

You may recall that the iconic "All in the Family" sitcom of the late 1970s starring Caroll O'Connor as Archie and Jean Stapleton as Edith, fearlessly addressed many taboo subjects. In a memorable episode, Archie, confounded by his wife Edith's newly irritable and aggressive personality, declared, "If it's the 'Change,' Edith, then change. On the count of three—one, two, three—CHANGE!"

Oh, Archie, if it were just that simple.

Menopause may send many of us into a tailspin, but it often sends our loved ones along with us. Our bodies act in new, bizarre ways. Families and friends may scratch their heads wondering where the cheerful, even-tempered person went and if she will ever return. A simple question like, "What's for dinner?" may elicit a volcanic blast where once upon a time, a simple shrug might have been the reply. Our emotional and mental states are adversely influenced by hormonal hell. This hormonal hell is physically apparent as well.

According to the *Association of Women for the Advancement of Research and Education Project,* there are 35 symptoms of menopause. Heading the list was hot flashes.

I've been at a conference table with a dozen, smart, articulate women of varying ages negotiating important programmatic, management decisions armed with facts, figures, and logic. Funny enough, the greatest dissension and constant discussion was the climate of the room. Some donned sweaters, others shed layers. Windows were opened and, immediately, rudely closed; the thermostat was lowered and, just as quickly, raised.

At one time in our lives *position* was everything—now it's climate! Amazingly, the outcomes from this meeting resulted in a streamlined, more efficient direction for the program, preservation of jobs, a reduction in expenses, and an increase in effectiveness—all in spite of the unrelenting climate drama.

Hot flashes aren't any fun during the day, but at night they can cause drama in the bedroom—and not the good kind. Awakening in a hot mess, thrashing about, and kicking off the covers are not conducive to our mates' sleep anymore than it is ours. Sleep itself is a hit or miss event during menopause. If by the grace of God one falls asleep, it's a sure thing by 3 a.m. you are wide awake staring at the ceiling. (Perhaps, all of us in this cycle of life should use this time to contact one another on social media?)

Another fun sidebar of menopause is the sprouting of facial hair: first a light shadow of a mustache and then prickly chin hairs that multiply as soon as they are plucked. Ironically, with this new growth of facial hair comes a marked decrease in hair "south of the border." I mean, really, one has to laugh at the contradictions of these happenings. Most women are annoyed with the facial sprouts, and others are almost as upset with being follicle-ly impaired below. One woman was so perturbed by the loss of the downy covering for her nether region that she treated herself to a tattoo where her hair line had been!

To add insult to injury, this time in our lives brings on new steps: *sneeze* cross your knees; *jump* tighten your thighs; *laugh* and it's all over! Nothing erodes self-confidence like incontinence.

However, once our periods end, and if our libido isn't too low, our vaginas not too dry, or our breasts too tender, we can become sexually active for the first time unconcerned with pregnancy. Hallelujah! Imagine no more pills or condoms (male or female).

Women will finally have the advantage over men of "Being ever ready." Men will be swallowing the little blue pill while we lustfully wait for it to kick in—which brings to mind that men have their own confrontation with life's changes; thus their acquisition of sports cars, toupees, and the arm candy of trophy wives as they struggle with aging as a fact of life. But, the male change is rarely spoken of and never with a capital "C."

I don't want arm candy, but I would gratefully trade in my all-wheel drive, grandma grocery-getter for a cougar, convertible coup! My four-wheel drive vehicle is useful in the Northeast. And, it is no coincidence that this is where I live, for I believe four seasons accurately describes our life cycle. I may now be in the winter of my life, but I fully intend it to be a very long, sunny winter with lots of indoor and outdoor games. When given the opportunity with a worthwhile gentleman, I will happily be *wined, dined,* and, on my word, *reclined.* Ahh! There are glories to menopause. It's not an end. It's a new beginning.

Menopause is a life-changing event but not the last women will experience. The symptoms are disconcerting and disruptive. But are they any more profound than the many other evolutions a woman experiences—from pre-school and adolescence through sexual activity, pregnancy, and motherhood just to name a few? Each new phase presents new physical, emotional, and cognitive challenges. Why do we in such a docile manner allow society's imposition of the capital "C" in "Change"?

I'm not belittling the impact this period (no pun intended) has on a woman's life. Rather, I'm applauding the knowledge and tools we have to help us negotiate it. Nutritionists and pharmacists have an ever-increasing arsenal to support biological normalcy. Prudent use of these tools with an empowered attitude and realization that our lives are just at another precipice will facilitate mental and emotional health. This change need not be threatening nor crippling; it can be another of life's natural progressions.

Learning Spanish to travel in Mexico so as to bring clothes and toys to indigent children. Graduation from college. Learning to sail on the Hudson River. Traveling solo cross country. Tap dancing. Attending a gourmet cooking school in Tuscany to learn to match wines with foods and to hunt truffles. These are just some of the things accomplished by postmenopausal women I know—each a life-changing event. But no capital "C" required.

I urge women to use the one tool always at their side: attitude. If we acknowledge menopause as a natural, unavoidable life progression, we can embrace it. It's not the enemy, just another part of whom we are and who we are becoming. We owe it to ourselves to deal with menopause in sane, concrete, and positive ways.

We owe it to our younger, female family members, colleagues, and friends to lead by example. How many of us were frightened by the "old wives' tales" of women having breakdowns brought on by the change, or their marriages destroyed by it? We can break this cycle by demonstrating our acceptance of the normalcy of this phase while addressing the physical and emotional challenges with available, appropriate remedies. They may not completely obliterate all the symptoms but can certainly make it an easier journey.

So open the windows, wear summer nightgowns, remember to smile when you feel like screaming, put sharp utensils away, see your doctor, and take advantage of all the help available. This change, like so many others, is only a beginning.

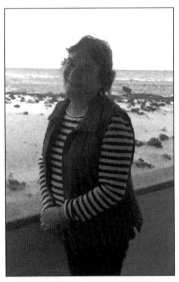

Grace Caddell is a woman, mother, grandmother, widow, Christian, friend, administrator, advocate for children and families, life-long learner, sometime writer and humorist, and post-menopausal. At sixty-four, writing a 100-word biography is daunting, so she began at the beginning. Raised in the Bronx, second child of five, she was nourished by the love of an extended family. Parochial schools engendered her desire to write and ignited her commitment to human services. Her husband empowered her to be better than she thought she could be. Her children and grandchildren encourage her pursuit of the next adventure in her life.

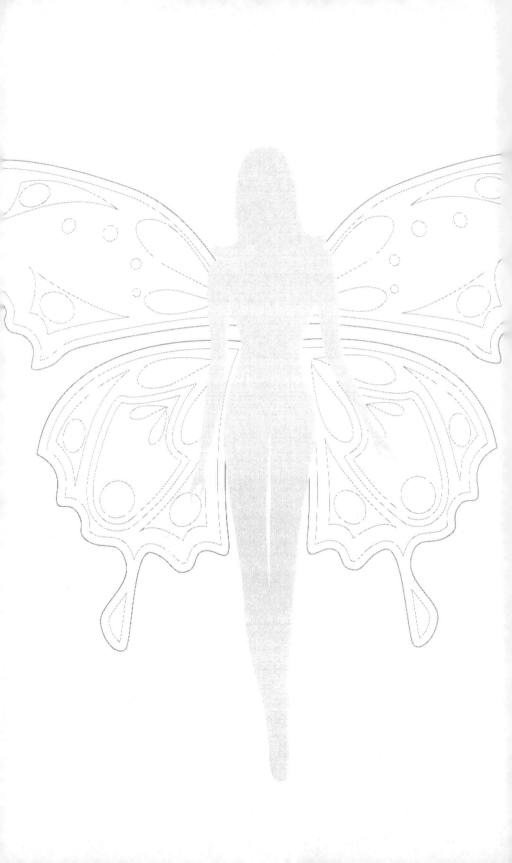

Cultivating Emotional Curiosity: Learning to Listen Beyond the Hormones

DR. JENEV CADDELL

Bob and Lisa sat on the small loveseat across from me in my cozy office, seemingly miles apart from each other. Bob crossed his legs away from Lisa, Lisa's upper lip was stiff, and both looked at me and away from me, appearing deflated and worn-out.

Finally, Lisa said, "We wanted to get some help for our marriage to see if we could make it work." She explained that she had been urging Bob to join her in couples counseling for years, but he was never the type of man to accept any type of help like that. It wasn't until Lisa suggested divorce that he finally came around.

"I just think people should be able to work things out for themselves," Bob said. "But if this is what she wants, I'm here, I'm open, I'm willing to see what it's like."

Such is the case for many couples. Nearly two decades of marriage and three kids later, they find themselves at a breaking point. One partner—in this case, Lisa—has felt an ever-painful distance, sometimes for years, making her feel invisible, unimportant, and frustrated. The more she tries to do something about it, the further her partner seems to disappear from her.

To Bob, however, his wife was a raging beast. No matter what he did, he couldn't please her. No matter what he said, it was never enough. He felt that his mere existence was enough to set off an attack.

He wanted to make Lisa happy, but he had no idea how. Any attempt he made was futile, just another reminder of how inadequate he was to her. So he stopped bothering. He became a pro at turning down the music when the symphony of frustration and disappointment began. He built up a wall to protect himself from her attacks and figured he was doing the relationship a favor by not contributing to the explosions.

Lisa got to the point where she could no longer take his distancing. Over the years, she figured that if she made herself loud enough, Bob would finally hear her. But it seemed like the opposite happened: The louder and angrier she got, the more he seemed to slip away, and the less he seemed to care. She had been shouting too much, and she felt ridiculous for trying to make herself seen to someone who, in her mind, obviously didn't want to see her. She started shutting down herself and giving up on her own expectations altogether.

This is when she knew something had to shift. Either they were going to figure this out together, or they were done. Getting outside help for their marriage was their only option.

At the heart of discontent in any marriage is an emotional disconnect. Neither partners feel important, valuable, or like a priority to each other, much less understood. A deep pain exists within each partner, yet neither see this within the other. It is often the case that each person rarely even understands the depth of his or her own experience, as few of us are cultured to be emotionally in touch and present with even ourselves.

Instead of feeling attuned with one's own emotional experience, partners have told me over the years that they have felt like they were losing their minds when disconnected from their other halves. They use life-and-death metaphors to describe how they feel in their relationships, and they feel crazy for making such a big deal of things. Add the hormonal fluctuations of menopause to the mix—adding fuel to the fire—and disconnected partners feel even more crazy.

What people aren't taught is that we actually *need* to be safely and securely emotionally connected with significant others in order to feel and be our best. Despite all of the praises of independence and autonomy, especially in western cultures, we are interdependent by nature. Individuals therefore begin to doubt themselves and start feeling crazy because of a natural biological response to separation and disconnect from their primary partners. The addition of the hormonal fluctuation that menopause contributes makes a woman's natural response to disconnect even harder to manage.

When we are disconnected from significant others in our lives, most notably our romantic partners, it does feel like a life-and-death matter. Even though we think we know better, we are still human, and our biology rules. When we are disconnected from our significant other, it's like we are cut off from the tribe. Evolutionarily speaking, that's tantamount to death. The brain spirals into a primal panic and sends danger signals to the rest of the body.

What we do with those danger signals depends on a few things, including how we were brought up as well as our natural temperaments. Many relationships are organized like Bob's and Lisa's in which one partner becomes frantic and loud, while the other distances himself and acts like it's no big deal, even though he's feeling flustered and inadequate.

A pattern then begins that is a recipe for disaster, one that psychologist Dr. John Gottman found led to divorce within five years if newly married couples get entrenched in it. The louder and angrier Lisa got, the further and further Bob moved away from her. The further that Bob moved away from her, the angrier Lisa got. Around and around they would go. Both partners showed each other the surface layer of their experience: Anger for Lisa, numbing out for Bob. Bob sees Lisa as a vindictive monster whom he can never please. Lisa sees Bob as a selfish, numbed-out iceberg who clearly doesn't care about her.

That's where my work as an Emotionally Focused Therapist and relationship coach comes in. Based on the latest science behind love, Emotionally Focused Therapy is the most rigorously researched form of couples counseling that has been proven to help nine out of ten couples improve their relationships. This approach to helping with couples works because it goes underneath the classic communication problems and surface issues and gets to the heart of the disconnect between partners: the emotional miss.

I helped Lisa and Bob repair their marriage from the inside out, largely using what I've learned about how love works, how couples lose each other, and how they can reconnect. I helped Lisa and Bob reach each other in a deeper way than they had even envisioned by helping them get out of the negative pattern they were caught in and start understanding each other.

It all started with each of them getting clear on what their deeper pain was all about. Bob knew that Lisa was angry with him. What he didn't know, and what Lisa didn't really even have a firm grasp of, was her experience at a deeper level. Similarly, Lisa knew that Bob would shut down and numb out, but she didn't realize how helpless and inadequate he felt as a husband. The emotional roller coaster in love is as turbulent as they come, but given that Lisa was experiencing hormonal fluctuations associated with menopause, it was even more challenging for her to navigate.

For anyone to get in touch with difficult emotions, it is necessary to slow everything down and be truly present, which is what Lisa and I did. We stayed together. I asked her to tell me about what was going on for her. With my hand gently holding hers as we walked down this dark abyss of primary emotions, she started to touch some of her feelings beneath the surface of her anger and frustration.

We stayed in a safe, accepting and curious space together, with Bob by her side, so that we could take a look at what was happening for her. She was able to untie the twisted knot of so many confusing feelings, and she began to articulate them. Her right emotional brain and left logical brain started having a conversation, which made her feel less out of control and more in her power.

I went through the same process with Bob, who was also able to touch deeper emotions that he hadn't even realized he was having. He explained he felt helpless and inadequate and he believed he could never be the man that she deserved. It wasn't that he didn't care; it was that he cared so much.

The real magic happens when couples are able to be present with their own deeper experiences, step away from the negative catch-22 cycle of escalating surface emotions, and let each other know what their true feelings are. Bob had no idea that underneath that fire-breathing dragon of his wife there was a scared and lonely woman desperate to connect with him. Similarly, Lisa had no clue that Bob just wanted to please her but felt like he never could. Learning this new information about each other was a rediscovery in its finest sense, and it shattered years of mistaken assumptions about each other that had only driven them apart.

Because "codependent" might be the dirtiest word of the first half of the 21st century, and few of us are raised to acknowledge how dependent we really are on each other, countless couples get caught up in a pattern similar to Bob and Lisa's. For one to fully be present with the deep and primal fear that accompanies an emotional disconnect with a spouse might feel like an acknowledgment of "weakness," in addition to being difficult to bear. Yet the truth is, the overwhelming emotional response that occurs is a natural response to help us do whatever we can to repair the bond. Far too often, the emotional response gets swept under the rug and we might try to think our way out of it. Then, as in the case of Bob and Lisa's, we start operating from surface emotions with each other, and we miss the big picture that we really matter to one another.

The bottom line is that partners really do matter to each other on a biological level, and our emotions clearly demonstrate that. We can't outthink our emotions. In the words of Dr. Sue Johnson, developer of Emotionally Focused Therapy, our emotions are the music to the dance of relationships. As Danielle LaPorte refers to them in her genius book *The Desire Map*, our emotions are the global positioning devices of our souls. Menopause might throw a few extra wrong turns and crazy roads on the map, but at the end of the day, our emotions are more important than we acknowledge.

The trick then, in and out of menopause, is to cultivate the art of fully being present, open, accepting and curious about our emotional experiences. When we do this, we listen to ourselves and use our emotions to guide us.

When something doesn't feel right in love, or in any part of life, pay attention to that feeling. Be open, accepting, curious, and present with it. This will empower you to be fully in touch with your experience so you can show up in the world fully integrated and self-aware. It then becomes that much easier to share these experiences with your partner, and when you can do this, you have a key to a healthy and strong relationship.

By going through the process on getting clear on their own emotional experiences, Bob and Lisa rediscovered themselves and each other. They re-prioritized their relationship and started showing up for each other in a way that no one had modeled for them before. Their kids were better off, they were both healthier and happier, divorce was no longer part of the discussion, and their marriage vows were renewed.

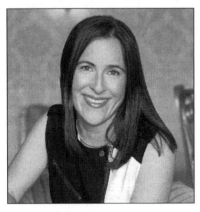

Dr. Jenev Caddell is a relationship coach and clinical psychologist who helps entrepreneurs and their partners communicate better, understand each other, and be happy together. She sees her work at the corner where the cutting-edge new science behind love meets business. Jenev understands that when we are stronger in love, we can do everything better. She believes that entrepreneurs are responsible for changing the world, and with rock solid relationships, they can do this even more effectively. Jenev is the author of Your Best Love: The Couples Workbook and Guide to Their Best Relationship *and founder of* www.MyBestRelationship.com.

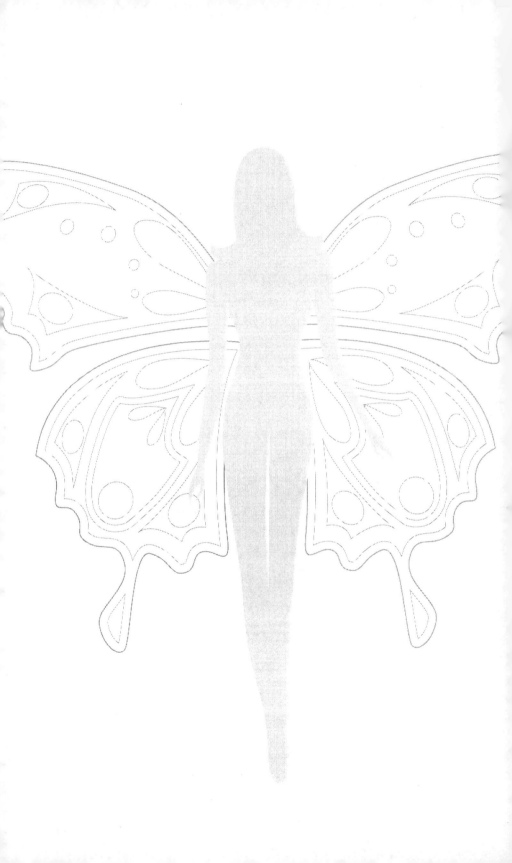

8

No One-Size-Fits-All Menopause

LINDA CELAURO

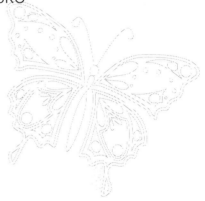

Finding out you're menopausal is pretty similar to getting your first period. The problem is nobody gives you a heads-up chat and a book. You don't get your ears pierced with a shiny pair of gold earrings and a sleepover with the girls to "celebrate."

I never even considered being menopausal because I never ever stopped to think about how old I was, not really! I didn't want to talk about it, didn't want to face the fact that I was nearing fifty.

But my body started doing things I just couldn't understand. I longed for the days I was able to fit into my clothes normally and not feel so unproportioned.

So I went to my gynecologist and was given a follicle-stimulating hormone (FSH) test. I was diagnosed with "ovarian insufficiency"—his words, not mine. In other words, perimenopause. Oh great! Within about three seconds, I started to feel old. Real old.

The magic number for my mom was forty-seven. Did I think I was immune? It's not like a "real" disease, right? It's a natural part of the life cycle to be lived through.

All these crazy thoughts started to run through my head. Perimenopause, what a stupid word. So I coined my own new word: menostart, the start of menopause, followed by menopause. And then there would be menopast—no more, your done, nadda nothing.

My doctor chimes in again, telling me 75 percent of women have menopause symptoms ranging from mild to severe. His recommendation was to have a bone density test, which I scheduled for the next week.

Suddenly, I had a flashback from the fifth grade when we had a back-to-school night for girls and mothers only. We watched the '60s flick "From Girl to Woman." My friends all eyeballed each other and cringed in our seats. The prepubescent chatter amongst us in school the next day was that Rhonda already had "gotten" hers.

Now I'm wondering why my own circle of friends wasn't really talking about the "change." So at the next one of our ladies luncheons, I brought up the subject. I always have to be the one with the initiative with this bunch—even though menopause may not be a hot topic of conversation during meals out.

Mary said she stopped about two years ago. She'd just never mentioned it. I had noticed her pants were getting very tight, but neither of us said anything. God forbid she has to go up a pant-size or two. Obviously, that extra weight is in no hurry to leave.

Lora said she was still going strong—you know just like clockwork every month with no end in sight.

Kathy—who is a few years older than the rest of us—got giggly, confessing that her granite kitchen countertop is her new best friend. During her hot flashes, it's her go-to remedy. She added those darn hot flashes wanted to turn her inside out.

Robin, a serial Internet dater, said she was a bit concerned when her last date pulled out a blue pill and guzzled it down with a cup of coffee.

Our conversation came to a halt at that moment as the busboy came over to refill our water glasses—and knocked one over, probably feeling nervous about overhearing our conversation. If I had to live through another one of Robin's dating stories, I just might lose my appetite for good!

Val, a high-end residential and commercial realtor on the Gold Coast of Long Island, confesses she has had lots of hot flashes. And, more than once she was meeting with a client when her hair went from styled to a curly ball of soaking wet.

The misconception amongst most of us is that hot flashes are over in a flash, Val says. No, they're long and come in stages. In the middle of the night, it's like global warming is happening right then and there, followed by a cooling down and a need to change sheets in the middle of the night. At least you no longer need a gym membership to break a sweat. It's like a gift that keeps on giving.

And it's my turn. Luckily for me, and my husband I might add, hot-flashes never played a major role. However, I severely have been suffering from insomnia. To this day, restful sleep eludes me. At least, I now have an excuse to say no to things I really don't want to do and blame it on the crushing fatigue. I did notice that once menopause hit, one of the first things to go was my brain. The brain that helped me coordinate school functions, business meetings, rehearsals, laundry, and bills no longer works quite the way it did—and I'll be the first to it admit it. At least I now have a really good use for all those sticky notes.

I realized from this gathering of my friends, there is no "one-size-fits-all" approach when it comes to menopause. It's an intimate issue so many women are uncomfortable sharing.

As I began my menopause journey, I went for my first bone density test. I felt good, looked good, and was a healthy weight for my height and body type. The not-so-good news was that I have osteopenia, a thinning of bone mass. While I did not have a necessarily severe case, it is considered to be a risk factor for the development of the more severe osteoporosis. I had a time-to-get-off-your-ass-bitch moment! It literally could have saved my life.

The positive that came out of this is that I realized I needed to start taking better care of me. After all, I deserve it.

Fast forward a bit: fifty-two when my periods finally stopped. Woo-hoo! No more half-opened tampon wrappers at the bottom of my handbag. Heck, I can even wear white again.

Come to think about it, maybe it *is* a cause for celebration. Sometimes, I can't actually decide. One day I embrace it, then, poof! It hits me right in the face. I can even get a tad bit grumpy about it. My roots are coming in; I hate taking time to get my hair colored, but unlike Jamie Lee Curtis, I don't have the complexion to rock gray.

As a Menopause Maven, we're at an age when we can save money on tampons, pads, pain relievers, and birth control pills and instead save for a great pair of Manolo Blahniks, maybe even a Birkin bag. Just the thought of this is making me happier. I think I may be on a roll now!

Do you want to hear the thing about menopause that surprised me most of all? For all the sleepless nights and the reluctance of those last few pounds to budge, I honestly feel like I really have gotten back some of that pre-adolescent freedom. The real thing about menopause that no one tells you is that life after the dreaded "change" can bring more balance, creativity, and self-acceptance than you ever dreamed possible.

Dealing with menopause and middle age issues does involve some suffering, some grieving and letting go.

But, despite all of the ups and downs, it's isn't all that bad. As women, we tend to be better at caring for others than ourselves. Be sure you're taking care of yourself with good food, exercise, and good health habits. In the long run, those healthy habits will ease this transition to this new part of life. Don't let menopause knock you out. With exercise, diet, symptom treatment, and great support, you can easily tackle this new life phase and look hot in a flash.

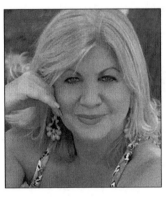

Linda Celauro is a leading expert in the field of Holistic Health and is the founder and owner of Savour Wellness LLC. She is a board certified integrative nutrition health coach, detoxification and weight loss expert, published author, and speaker. She has trained in practical lifestyle management techniques and innovative coaching methods with some of the world's top health and wellness experts. A member of the International Association for Health Coaches and the American Association of Drugless Practitioners, Linda is an active participant in several health coach communities.

Her passion for holistic medicine stems from her own personal health struggles and life experiences. After spending twenty years as a busy professional in a

Fortune 500 company, she found herself sick and burned out. Upon leaving her job, she spent years of studying, obtaining multiple certifications and transforming her life. Using food as medicine, she unlocked the keys to vibrant health and wellness. Linda is deeply passionate about inspiring others to reclaim their vitality and health. She helps people reach their health and wellness goals by offering in-person and online assistance with weight loss and clean-eating protocols.

Her first book, Healthy Eating Manifesto, was published in 2014. She is also a contributing writer to several well known health publications. She also serves on the advisory board for www.theglam.net (green living and media network). Linda is proud to be a contributing author to Menopause Mavens: Master the Mystery of Menopause. Linda's all new program, No Sweat to Sexy, Svelte and Shapely and more "hot" topics about menopause are available at *www.HotInAFlash.com.*

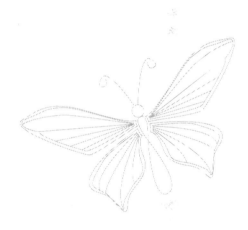

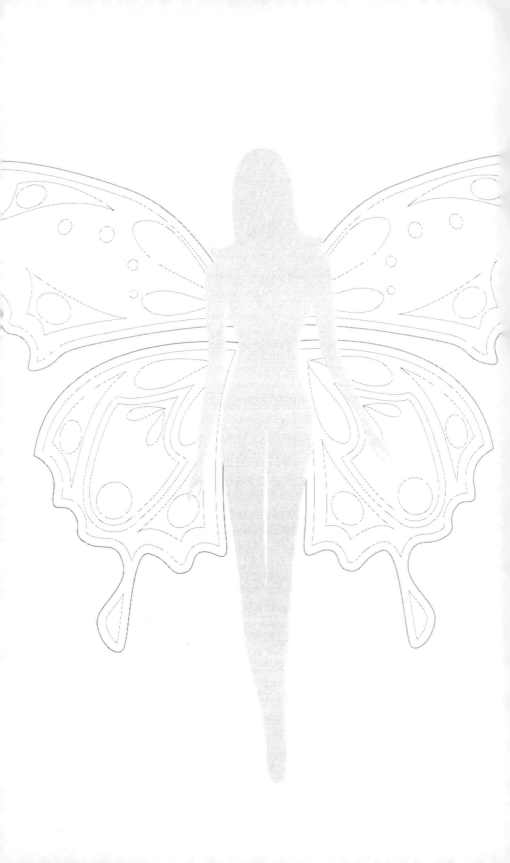

9

Embodying the Dragon: The Great Power Surge!

KATIA COOPER

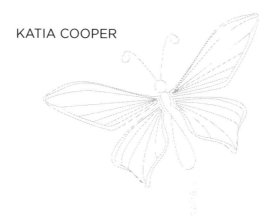

"Dragon: Kundalini power. Fire from dragon purifies negative thinking, dispels illusion. Slaying the dragon means confronting and eliminating fears, enabling yourself to awaken higher level of awareness."

—Betty Bethards, *The Dream Book Symbols for Self-Understanding*

In my life, "the change" has been about slaying what is not serving the greater good—and using its influence to awaken an advanced state of consciousness. The wisdom that develops through perimenopause and menopause can identify what is precious now and release what is no longer needed.

My indicators of menopause have manifested as tension, anxiety, tightness, pain, hot flashes, and distraction from the present. However, when I listen to the inner signs of what the symptoms are trying to tell me, menopause has a clarity and precision. This stage in life seems to have secret codes that, once cracked, can make life simpler. As I have reclaimed more authenticity and deepened into my Wise Self, it is as if I have become privy to understand more of the mysteries and how to play. It all starts with curiosity and patient consideration.

Some questions to ask: How do I embody the power of dragon fire without harming what is valuable to me? How do I choreograph my dance through life, accessing love, power, and both my feminine creativity and my masculine drive to respond and relate in the most fulfilling ways?

For me, dancing takes me toward the answer. When I dance and embody the energy of flow and power, I receive insight that guides me in my inner and outer life. The gift of moving physically in this way is that my intention brings change at a very grounded level and integrates it into the other realms of mind, spirit, and emotions.

ENTER THE DRAGON: PERIMENOPAUSE

At age forty-seven, I was blessed with practicing "the art of living," which included consciously "moving my body for pleasure." These were only two of the many brilliant concepts I learned through The Nia Technique. Nia is a playful fitness dance class that engages participants to connect to the four personal realms—body, mind, emotion, and spirit—as well as to the group in a wildly fun and transformative way. It also offers much more than that—a magical portal into our potential. My Nia practice and teaching enhanced my lifestyle and ultimately became a lifesaver when some devastating challenges arose.

In perimenopause, I was dedicated to doing what could best support me and my service to the world. I was juggling my creative endeavors, including my insightful work as a Reiki Master and Teacher. At age forty, I had made a firm commitment to "Mastery"— or Self-Mastery—a challenge to continue my best personal growth. Over the years, I had dealt with a lot of self-healing, both alone and with the help of other wonderful practitioners. I attribute my gift as a healer to a high level of sensitivity and inner spirituality that, for many years, I had hid out of a sense of self-doubt. I learned how to listen, honor, and engage Spirit with my gifts from an extraordinary and enlightened teacher, Nancy Retzlaff. I affectionately referred to her as my Spiritual Mother.

As I approached perimenopause, a sense of confidence and ful-fillment was mounting for me, way beyond what I had known. Life had reached a moderately consistent high for me. I was steeped in gratitude, sharing the loves of my life—dancing for the joy of it and offering intuitive healing sessions.

This stable space, along with the fervor of perimenopause brought me closer to discovering buried, unspeakable ordeals from long ago.

A few months into some very intense bodywork, coupled with psychotherapy, repressed memories of sexual abuse from my very early childhood arose. I felt like I was falling inside a tumultuous trap, like the rabbit hole that Alice stumbled into, only with extended horror. The pedophile was someone my parents knew well. In the company of adults, he appeared shy and socially inept, with a pre-tentious smile. The truth is, he was deeply disturbed, and terribly violent, acting out as a monster to children who were preschool age and younger.

I wanted to "get past" each memory, so quickly that I scanned over the devastation of my inner child with unrealistic expectations and more denial of how deep the open wounds of utter terror went. This only caused post-traumatic stress disorder (PTSD) to erupt with stronger memories and emotions. Nightmares kept me from sleeping, rendering me more vulnerable to re-experience what was horrifically vicious. I felt like I was being emotionally hijacked by my infant, toddler, and very young child in their desperate need to get help from me. I had a lot to learn to become present to the intensity for my innermost victim.

So I did my internal work to the point of exhaustion. At times, I had the energy to seek help. The PTSD that had been neglected for more than forty-six years did not give in to logic. Its turmoil fought to get the attention that had been overdue for a lifetime.

AN EPIC JOURNEY

While I was exasperated with the length of my recovery, an idea came to me and I was finally able to find meaning for all the time I spent. I discovered freedom by surrendering to my intention to provide all the love and nurturing my inner self needed, no matter how long it would take. Granting this was only fair, to make up for all my losses. I had suffered the emotional abandonment of caretakers, especially my parents' protection and validation of my experiences and feelings. Due to the lack of verbal and mental abilities in my first five years of life, the invalidation of my story by adults made me think I was crazy. Subconsciously, this made me question my rationality anytime another opposed my view. The truth of questioning my sanity was not about "my craziness" but the temporary insanity of adults who lacked ability to be responsible for a child and the repercussions of denying that harm.

As I tended to the depth of my own healing, I wished that no child would ever experience this type of absurd abuse. As I continued to offer my healing services and movement classes, I discovered that many others had been burdened by the secrecy of childhood sexual abuse. I began collecting a medley of resources to help survivors of sexual abuse and began writing my own books to help lift the shame and energetically recover the lightness and authentic spirit that gets buried in the survivor.

EMBRACING THE DRAGON

Out of the torment of abuse, re-traumatization, and the arduous work of therapy came a deep, resilient desire to create ways to make the recovery work lighter. My Nia dance practice and the creative genius—recovered inner child—gave me the tools to create that lightness. Many times, I succeeded in lessening my emotional pain by consciously moving my body, choosing more pleasure through each movement. Emotions held in my cells could unwind as I chose more joy in each body activity.

In a healing process, seeking pleasure means moving in the direction that diminishes pain, in order to shift toward a lighter state of being. The "creative genius" brought deep insight and resolution through delightful fairy tales and the undertaking of sharing them through books.

My mastery in menopause has been about clearly standing in my truth and reclaiming what was taken from me. The energy of menopause and claiming my wisdom moves me to continue taking steps to regain all the joy, the innocence, the love, the personal rights, and the confidence that would have grown in me had I not been violated in my formative years. I keep opening to receive what a child of the Divine deserves, creating new neuropathways for love and abundance to flow.

EMBODYING THE DRAGON

Now, when I feel a hot flash or power surge coming on, I ask myself, "How can I recognize all of my power?" Sometimes as I feel into that power, I tremble subtly with humbleness and awe at what I sense inside as a connection with the Divine. The more I allow space for that energy, the more I enjoy experiences such as the crown of my head energizing like a large funnel gently widening beyond the circumference of my skull. Often, the top of my head is tingling in anticipation as calm waves of love enter my body for longer periods of time. I am grateful beyond words, to Source, our Creator, and for all who have helped to bring me to this place of self-love that allows me to share greater compassion, vision, and potential for mankind to evolve.

My dragon fire power is not power over another. It is an empowerment from within that holds the energy of what I need, whether it's healing, slowing down, or trusting my intuition and the Universe; it is strength, courage, compassion, or confidence beyond my usual limits.

As I discover ways to harness my power, I realize the unlimited potential of the Divine. I recognize the infinite gifts that Source energy offers, as well as the responsibility I have to regulate my life force—to not overload or shut down—for long-term wellness. Imagine the attention to detail it takes to be an electrician. Then, imagine the steps of becoming a master electrician and all the different applications to channel the energy most proficiently. I believe the integration of our own energy mastery is what gives each us the most fulfillment as we continue to grow into our own Wise Woman.

I have to admit that I resist expanded power at times, in my illusion to get more done. That is when hot flashes get most intense, urging me to release my habit of "trying too hard." I am still learning to surrender and recognize the gift of embodying the Wise Sage in me. I welcome her deeper as I join in this group of highly perceptive authors, my Maven Sisters. It almost takes my breath away to recognize the security and foundation of consciousness we are holding for this Right of Passage for upcoming Crones of Light. May we all shine our truth for every crone in the making—that she may find her way in the purification process of menopause, purposefully using her own inherent dragon fire power to celebrate the most spiritually connected time of life!

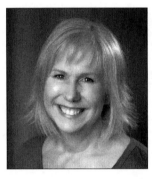

Katia Cooper is an author, a facilitator for dance and healing workshops, and a Reiki Master/Teacher. Her metaphysical training, research, and practices span almost four decades. Katia's healing work gently taps into the subconscious to bring buried wounds to the Divine Light. She plans to publish a series of books— Heart and Sole Journey . . . . an Elf's Healing Story from Sexual Abuse—*to share creative and even delightful paths of reclaiming wholeness for teen and adult survivors of childhood abuse. Katia experiences many beings shifting consciousness by coming* into personal power—changing old patterns into a safer future for children.

Learn more: **www.KatiaCooper.com**

10

My Awakening to the Divine Feminine

MICHELE GITA DAISH

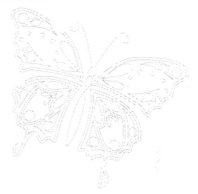

My entrance into perimenopause began just after my thirty-sixth birthday. I would awaken in the middle of the night, swimming in sweat as if I had just stepped out the shower. My bed sheets and night clothes were cold and wet, soaked to the bone. Some nights, I had to change the bed because it was too cold and wet to sleep and my mattress was soaked through. Every night I had to change my clothes. At first, I was alarmed and wondered if the bed clothing was too heavy, so I lightened my side of the bed, placing a very thin blanket on me, while my husband slept next to me bundled inside a thick comforter.

It took me several years to realize that I was actively in peri-menopause. I was in denial about it. After all, I was only thirty-six years old, vibrant, and at my supposed sexual peak as a woman in my late-thirties. I still had my menstrual cycle every twenty-eight days like clockwork for the next thirteen years. And then my peri-menopausal symptoms gradually began to amplify after my forty-second birthday.

Sleeping through the night was no longer possible as my hor-mones were completely out of whack—insomnia, hot flashes, and migraine headaches were constant. I took to sleeping on the couch downstairs so I wouldn't bother my husband. I was tired, agitated, angry, and annoyed. I felt betrayed by my body. I saw an acupuncturist twice a month to ease my symptoms, and I took herbal remedies.

My first period at age twelve is as vivid a memory as menopause. I had entered into womanhood with whispers and traces of blood, tiny spotting and marks on my cotton underwear. I wondered what it was and asked my mother. She bought me a box of Kotex pads and a belt, and with no further explanation, said I would need to learn to live with this for many years. I recall feeling so grown up. I was still a kid inside, and yet my womanhood was being born. I had an older sister who had not yet reached menarche and two younger sisters who were far away from starting their own cycles, so I was truly on my own figuring this out.

I've had epilepsy since age twelve, too. My seizures occurred often during the early phases of my menses into my mid-twenties. When I became pregnant with my daughter at age twenty-nine, I had no seizures, and it seemed pregnancy hormones agreed with me. I had a daughter, and, ten months later, had a son. My marriage could not withstand the birth of two babies within a year, and we divorced when our son was six months old, after less than three years of marriage. I was a single mother raising two toddlers, ages three and four, when I met my future husband Michael two years later—he had a four-year old. Twenty-five years later, we are still together.

I've always sought spirituality, and my seeking intensified in my early forties as I fully entered menopause. My hormones were completely out of whack and my seizures had worsened to the point that I underwent a week-long hospitalization and brain study in an effort to locate where the seizures were occurring in my brain. Anti-seizure medications were not working for me, and I had uncontrolled seizures, causing me to seek alternatives to medication. I had a surgical implant placed into my chest leading into my neck and brain. At forty-five years old, I was still a few years away from entering menopause. I remember being unable to move my head and neck, sitting with a huge bandage on my neck—but I went to church anyway. I prayed for a miracle. I knew I had been close to death on more than one occasion, and I knew that my surgery would forever change me. Now, I live with an implanted device in my body, and I've had it replaced twice.

I began to question my reason for being alive. I had nearly drowned when my children were seven and eight years old when I had a seizure in a swimming pool and floated to the bottom of a twelve-foot pool. Grace intervened in the form of two teenage girls who saved me from drowning. The summer of my near-drowning incident, my husband and I would lay awake night after night talking, wondering how we would cope if one of us died. Searching for my purpose for being on this earth, I deeply immersed myself in the study of spirituality and world religions in an effort to understand the world's creation and my place in it.

As I entered the final phase of menopause, I also entered a seminary program and spent four years immersing myself in the study of creation from the aspect of the seven major world religions. I deeply studied the yoga sutras and kriya yoga, the philosophical branch of yoga, and became a disciple of an enlightened teacher.

These final days of menopause were just as grace-filled as those early days at age twelve. I knew when I had my last period that it would be my last. It left as quietly as it arrived. It was only a couple of days of spotting, light and clear. My cycle ended the same way it began. I was entering a new chapter of my life, and I chose to embrace it full on, with grace and vitality.

After graduating from seminary, I completed a 200-hour yoga teacher training. I began teaching yoga, and completed my studies at Institute of Integrative Nutrition. Now I understand my unique purpose for being born, my *Sva Dharma*. I was here to help others— to be a vehicle for their transformation. My life's work is to teach meditation, yoga, and healthy lifestyle principles to others. I am an Awakener, a "guide-on-the-side," teaching others who they are and that they can truly know themselves as unique souls born into this world with gifts to share with the world.

I'm fortunate to have experienced very little womanly distress during the thirty-nine years of my menstrual cycle. Even though I had migraine headaches and seizures during the worst years, the best years gave me two easy, stress-free pregnancies and two healthy babies.

The monthly bloating, bleeding, and cramps somehow bind women together in sisterhood. We discuss our cramps and bloating like badges of honor, youth, and fertility.

Yet, how do we keep the sisterhood alive *after* menopause as the vibrancy of youth leaves us?

I came into my true power as a fully grown woman when I entered my final years of menopause. I now know that these are the years women can speak their truth, own who they are, learn why they are here, and clean up their pasts. I have learned to deeply care for myself so I can care for others. The "pause" is a time of illumination, introspection, knowing, choice, and discovery.

My biggest challenge as a postmenopausal woman is allowing myself to age with grace and ease, not falling into societal pressure to look younger. As I look in the mirror and see lines, wrinkles, and age spots, I remind myself that the gift of youth is ours but for a short time. Maturity and grace are gifts to us as we go through life's challenges.

With age comes wisdom. With wisdom comes freedom.

As you approach menopause, perhaps it would benefit you to explore the questions below for yourself. Take time to journal, reflect, and meditate. The answers are within you if you quiet your mind and listen to your soul. Answering these questions can provide a launching board for you to propel yourself into the next chapter of your life:

What vision wants to be birthed by me at this stage of my life?

How can I identify myself beyond mother/wife/daughter/sister/ businesswoman?

What unique skills, traits, and gifts are mine to share?

What do I need to accept about my life at the end of my reproductive cycle?

Spending time exploring these questions can provide important indicators of what's next for you. How you choose to spend your postmenopausal years is up to you. Create what you want to be. You have the power; you've always had it! Menopause can be the time to discover for yourself just how powerful you are.

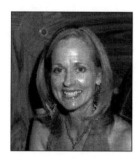

Michelle Gita Daish *is a certified holistic health coach, a registered yoga instructor, and a San Francisco Bay Area native.*

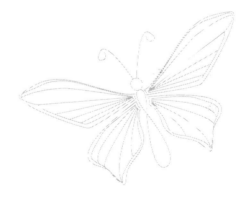

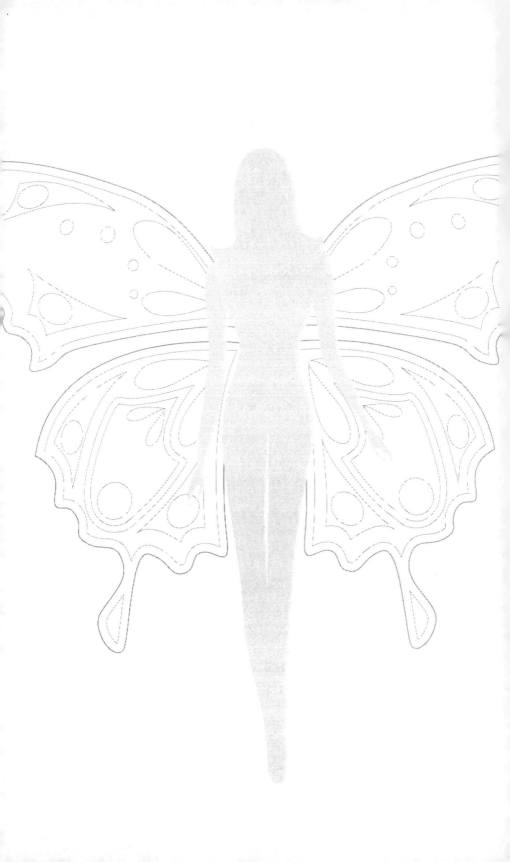

11

Hand Over the Chocolate and No One Gets Hurt!

DONNA DAVIS

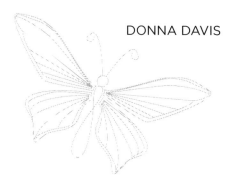

Menopause can be dangerous—no *ifs*, *ands*, or *buts* about it. This is not something that should be taken lightly, although a healthy sense of humor—and chocolate, of course—can help get you through it.

It's a rather interesting time in a woman's life with so much happening in your brain, your body, and your world. Each and every day can pose a new, often unexpected twist or turn of mood, seemingly uncontrollable emotions, and, many times, completely irrational behavior and/or reactions that can lead to utter chaos. It can also happen in record time—in split seconds, in fact, with no warning!

There is no official survivors' guide, yet I humbly offer these suggestions both for yourself and others.

SOME DO'S AND DON'TS OF BEING NEAR A MENOPAUSAL WOMAN

<u>Don't</u> try to talk me off the edge. Chances are, if you're in my vicinity you now become my prisoner and are coming with me when I go over.

<u>DO</u>: Kindly offer me chocolate and walk away. (Save yourself.)

Don't tell me it's okay or that it will be. It's not, and how the hell do you know anyway? Do you have some magic crystal ball that solves all woes?

DO: Just keep your mouth shut and give me chocolate! (Seems easy enough.)

Don't tell me to relax and breath. Oh, I'm breathing all right. I'm breathing fire, and unless you want your ass burnt to a crisp, I suggest you steer clear of me and walk the other way, pretend you don't even see me. Eye contact can be dangerous!

DO: Chocolate will do just fine, thank you. (Can you handle that?)

Don't tell me you understand. Chances are you don't even have a friggin' clue! You might have a general idea or smidgen of understanding if you are in your forties or older. But, yeah, you guessed it....

Do: HAND OVER THE CHOCOLATE AND NO ONE GETS HURT! (Let's keep this simple.)

Now I want to be clear. It is not the woman that is the savage beast; it is her hormones, the lack of them, actually, or the hormones trying to figure out exactly what their exit strategy is. This time in a woman's life is certainly serious business. There are many things going on—often in several different directions. A woman may need to reach out to girlfriends who have gone through menopause already, as well as trained medical professionals to help ease the process.

Along with professional help, I advocate strongly for the chocolate experience.

Chocolate goes well with *everything*. There are endless varieties, too! You can enjoy something different every single day. I bet you can consume a different piece of chocolate every day of the year and never have the same piece twice—365 days of chocolate… ahhh… can you imagine it?

You can eat it anywhere, or, more accurately, *everywhere!* You can be home in your sweats, driving down the highway, outside while walking the dog, at the beach, or in the boardroom. You can even have some during a hot flash; melted chocolate is wonderful!

You can eat it *anytime!* Day or night, or the minute you wake up (if you managed to sleep). It's a wonderful meal or meal substitute. An afternoon snack, or perhaps an appetizer for each and every meal (my personal favorite). Of course you can have it for dessert like ordinary folks, but why limit yourself?

After consuming endless pieces of chocolate, resulting in somewhat of a caffeine high and temporarily ensuring the safety of others, you may realize that you consumed a gazillion calories. This may trigger the sadness and guilt response that puts you in a spin cycle of thinking, "How the hell will this belly fat come off?" or "Why did I let myself get so out of control?" or "How did I jump two dress sizes?" or "Whose hips are these, anyway?" Be kind to yourself. You are going through a rough time and it's okay. Chocolate may very well be your best friend during a time like this. You can get through this together.

As far as exercise goes, the jury is still out on that one. Some people swear by it, others curse it! One size certainly does not fit all. We each have our own trials, successes, failures, and options. Good luck with that. I'll stick with chocolate.

THE ULTIMATE OBSTACLE COURSE

Menopause should be considered an Olympic sport. After all, it's very similar to an obstacle course.

Competitions can include:

- How much sleep can you lose in one night? Or better yet a week, a month, a year?
- How many seconds does it take to get from calm to crazy? This one may need a photo finish.

- Rating the severity of a hot flash. Who can reach the highest temperature without combusting?
- How many boxes of tissues does it take to get through a rough day?
- How many chocolate candy bars can you consume in three minutes?
- Did I say that out loud? How many ways can you verbally cut, slice and dice someone? (Spectators should bring earplugs.)
- How many swears can you say in one sentence? (The person with the most bleeped out words wins!)

THE DRIVING CHALLENGE:

The driver from Team A has a passenger in the car from Team B. Have Driver A successfully complete the course without Passenger B vomiting, wetting her pants, grabbing the wheel, or ejecting herself from the car. Can you imagine? You need nerves of steel—and a good bladder—for this test!

Prizes may include but not be limited to:
- A suitcase full of chocolate: at least 365 pieces—one for each day of the year (although it really won't last that long).
- A year's supply of tissues: at least 52 boxes of pretty, soft, strong ones.
- A month's supply of sheets: 31 complete sets so you can change your sheets at least once a night.
- A year's supply of laundry detergent to wash all those sheets and the countless other clothes that get drenched during your hot flashes.
- A year's worth of car insurance with the highest amount of coverage possible.

Menopause can also be considered a COMBAT sport.

Scenario 1: Menopausal woman (MW) goes to the checkout counter. The cashier barely acknowledges her (if she's lucky) because she is having a conversation with a co-worker about the latest gossip or what the plans are for this weekend.
Does she:

    A. Sarcastically say, "I'll wait until you're done with your conversation, then you can do your job and help me."

    B. Say, "Are you both working? Does your manager know that you are not taking care of customers because your personal conversation is more important?"

    C. Walk out of the store in a rage because of the lack of service and respect?

    D. All of the above.

Scenario 2: MW realizes that everyone on the road is an idiot! Where did they all come from!? Were they always here and she just didn't notice?
Does she:

    A. Justifiably beep at the person who has had their blinker on for the last 2 miles until they shut it off?

    B. Weave around several cars and turn on red simply because the light is taking too damn long?

    C. As a result of all the traffic, become furious because no one knows how to drive and now are all in her way?

    D. Want to get out of her car and cause serious bodily harm to the person who dared to beep at *her*?

    E. All of the above.

Scenario 3: MW comes to the conclusion that *nothing* makes sense and *everything* irritates her to no end!
Does she:

A. Wonder why her co-workers/staff make such asinine decisions and fusses under her breath along with displaying facial contortions that express her disgust?

B. Simply not comprehend or understand the laziness of each and every individual in the household and want to scream at them?

C. Become deeply grateful that no one can read her mind or hear her thoughts because she could be slapped, beaten, fired, or jailed?

D. Feel like no one on the face of the earth exhibits any common sense whatsoever and she secretly wishes to beat it into every last one of them?

E. All of the above!

Like I said, menopause can be dangerous!

Life is too short. Chocolate is a wonderful tool to help you through the dark days of menopause (or any day for that matter) and back into the light of your life.

So when in doubt, eat the chocolate! Haven't you heard? It fixes *everything!*

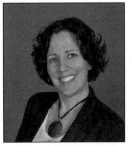

Donna Davis, a life-long resident of New Jersey, has been an educator, teacher, and nanny for 30 years, using humor as a teaching tool. She cherishes the journey of life and loves — you guessed it — chocolate.

Learn more: ***www.theMenopauseFairy.com***

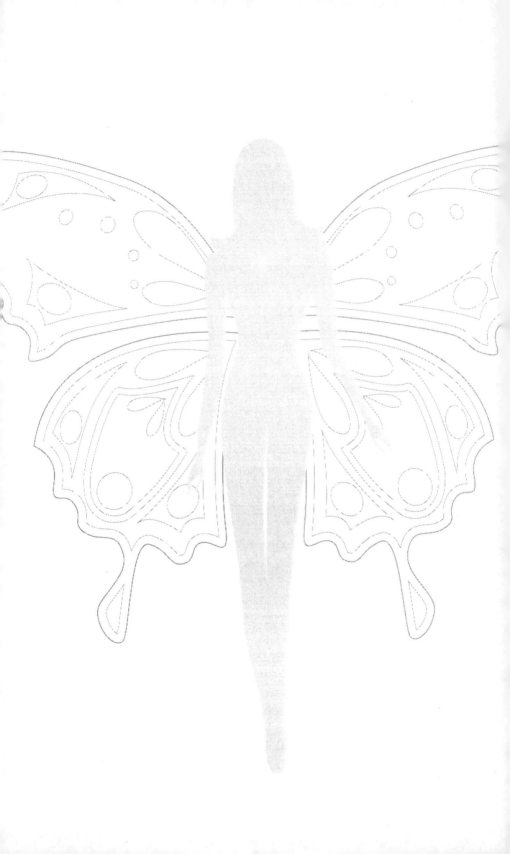

12

How to Work with Your Health Care Provider to Get the Care You Deserve

ANNA D. GARRETT, PHARMD, BCPS, CIC

I've had it.

Had it with hearing how my clients are dismissed by their health care providers for being "too young" to be in perimenopause.

For being "too far past menopause" to have hormonal symptoms.

When I was in pharmacy school and we had our pain management lectures, we were taught that "pain is what the patient says it is." And while I'm not managing pain with my clients (though you'd be amazed at what cutting out gluten and dairy can do), the principle is the same. Hormone issues are whatever the client says they are!

Part of the problem with quick dismissals by care providers relates to how the system is set up. Your average garden-variety physician has to see a patient every seven minutes if he or she wants to maintain a certain level of income. Productivity requirements have killed the doctor-patient relationship in many ways. Who has the time to get to the bottom of an issue that can be Band-Aided with an antidepressant or birth control pills?

The other large piece of this is that most physicians get, at best, surface level training in dealing with hormonal problems in menopause. Any MD that has more than this level of knowledge has sought that out independently. But it's tough to work in extra training when the revolving door of patients never stops.

A growing number of hormone specialists in the United States are operating "wellness clinics." These practices cater to cash-paying women who want hormone replacement. And they make a big chunk of their profit by inserting hormone pellets in the butts of these women. Which is fine for our sisters who choose to go that route.

But what about the "hormone hesitant" among us?

I am one of these women. My family tree has breast or uterine cancer on every branch of it.

Both grandmothers.

My mother.

My sister (at age forty!).

I feel like I have a big red target on my back. But I'm very blessed to have been spared at this point. There's not a doctor under the sun who would responsibly write me a prescription for estrogen.

When I decided to create my business, I wanted to work with women who were looking for alternative solutions. That's where my expertise as a pharmacist comes in very handy! Many people think pharmacists only know about prescription drugs.

Au contraire!

In our six years of training, we are also taught about herbs, vitamins, and other natural alternatives. For me, this was the perfect marriage of my years of training and my desire to serve women who were like me.

Not only am I passionate about creating management plans, for my ladies, I'm also fired up about teaching women how to advocate on their own behalf in a somewhat broken health care system. As a pharmacist, I know I get treated differently by providers because I know what questions to ask and have already done my research. That's one of the perks of being in school forever!

But what about the rest of the world? How do you develop confidence and muster up the courage to have a voice and get your needs met?

I've put together this list of eleven steps to help you start building confidence. The courage? Well, that just takes practice and requires a willingness to hang tough knowing that your health depends on it.

1. **Above all else, trust that you know your body better than anyone.** Never forget this. Even if your provider says "it's all in your head." Your body has innate wisdom that only you are aware of. Trust that wisdom and keep searching for the right caregiver until you find someone who is willing to listen and respects your point of view.

2. **Ask yourself high-quality questions when it comes to your health.** "Will my insurance pay for this?" isn't one of them. High-quality questions include:

   - What is the return on my investment if I do XYZ?
   - How will feeling better impact my life?
   - What's it costing me to do nothing?
   - Do I *really* want my insurance company deciding how good I can feel?

3. **When you meet with your provider, be organized and to the point.** Prioritize your questions and concerns and address those first.

4. **Take an active role in your care.** A "doctor knows best" attitude will not serve you. At all. If your doctor is impatient or rushes you, start looking for another one.

5. **Do a little preliminary research about your symptoms.** Perimenopause has at least 34 symptoms, so you can't rely on your BFF's experience to mimic your own.

   Know a little bit about what your options are and what you want for yourself.

   - Hormones or no?
   - Willing to make big lifestyle changes or no?
   - Antidepressants or no?
   - Sleeping pills or no?

The more clarity you have here, the better able your provider will be to make helpful recommendations. And don't be afraid to say no if things are going in a direction you don't like. **Remember, you are in charge!**

6. **Consider working with an alternative provider.** Most people wouldn't think about working with a Doctor of Pharmacy to get their hormones balanced. But I offer testing, customized management plans and lots of hand holding. No, your insurance probably won't cover working with me, but what's it costing you to do nothing? Plus, I'll give you a level of care that you can't possibly get in a seven-minute visit.

   Other helpful alternative care providers include acupuncturists (great for hot flashes), massage therapists, naturopaths, and herbalists.

7. **Don't downplay any symptoms or physical complaints you may have.** All too often, when you're sitting in a doctor's office, you get an attack of the "it's not really that bad" syndrome and either don't mention problems you've been having or mention them as an afterthought, as if it's really not a big deal.

   Embarrassed by whatever is going on? Trust me; most providers have seen and heard it all if they've been in practice for more than a minute. The bottom line is that your doctor won't be able to help you if you don't clearly and honestly present any physical complaints. Do her and yourself a favor by speaking up (this is where the courage part comes in). A confident patient who is upfront about what's going on gets the best care.

8. **Be sure you understand the doctor's answers and don't be afraid to ask for further explanations.** Just because your doctor *thinks* she's answered your questions doesn't necessarily mean she has. If your doctor explains something to you but you're still unclear about it simply say so and ask for further explanation. Don't go home and wonder (or call later and get stuck in phone tree hell).

9. **Asking follow-up questions at the right time saves time for both you and the doctor.** Get information in writing. People remember less than half of what is told to them in a visit. And with the menopausal crowd, it's probably less than that. I speak from experience.

10. **If you're confused, ask for information in people-speak, not medical-ese.** Often a doctor will tell you about procedures or treatments using high falutin' technical language . . . and you have only the vaguest idea of what she's talking about. Speak up!

    Ask for a translation in simple, layperson's terms. If you don't understand what is being said, you can't make educated decisions.

11. **Once you and your provider have decided on a course of action, keep up your end of the deal.** There are few things more frustrating from my standpoint as a care provider than creating an elegant management plan for my client only to have them do nothing.

    - Can't afford the meds? Say so before leaving.
    - Do the instructions sound overwhelming? Ask your provider to start with a smaller management step.
    - Have no desire to make lifestyle changes? Be honest and say so.

Your health care provider is in practice because she wants you to rock your mojo! Good communication skills are an important piece of this. But let's face it; sometimes it's just not a good fit and it's time to break up. Here's how to skillfully navigate *that*.

The least mature way to leave your doctor is the sneak attack. This is when you sign a medical records release form and skedaddle. A more grown-up way (which increases confidence and courage) is to talk with your doctor about why you're not clicking. Don't just run away and leave, because maybe something can be salvaged.

Managing menopause is a big job. It takes a village. Give careful thought and consideration to the people you put on your team. After all, they're going to help you become a rockin' old lady. Your health-care providers are an integral part of that team—at least as important as your hairdresser or your trainer, right? Remember, you're in charge of your health 24/7 and you will always be your own best advocate.

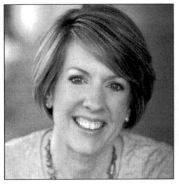

Dr. Anna D. Garrett has been a clinical pharmacist for more than twenty years and has worked in a variety of practice settings. She is a Doctor of Pharmacy and Board Certified Pharmacotherapy Specialist. She is also a Certified Intrinsic Coach® and has studied through the American Academy of Anti-Aging Medicine. While traveling her career path, Dr. Garrett discovered that working with women in midlife is her true passion. Dr. Garrett is passionate about teaching women how to navigate the sometimes-choppy waters of this transition. She offers a variety of services including hormone balancing, weight loss coaching, and health coaching for women in perimenopause and menopause.

*Learn more: **www.drannagarrett.com***
*Email: **info@drannagarrett.com***

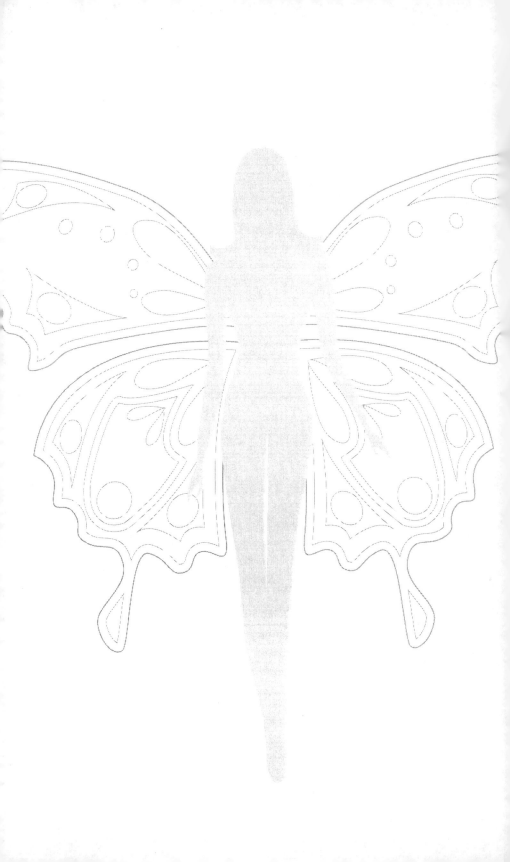

13

How My Ovaries Ran My Life

MEREDITH KRIEBEL

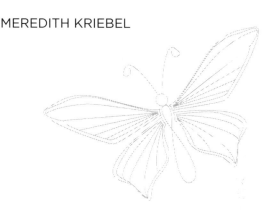

At thirty-six, I was in the midst of grad school. It was a brutal academic experience. I felt beaten financially, socially, and emotionally. I did it because it seemed like the right thing to do. I had always said I wanted a master's … in anything. I don't even know why. Arbitrary. People wanted me to have goals, and here I was in a doctorate program. It was hideous but everyone was proud of me.

What I really wanted, in retrospect, was to get laid as much as possible. I wanted every kind of kinky dirty sex I could get. If I could have figured out how to make it a respectable past-time or job, I would have. I wish someone had given me permission. I was trying to be some version of moral and respectable that seemed appropriate. Don't get me wrong! I was a liberated queer advocate fiend all about consent and getting what you need in a safe, sane and responsible way. There was just enough cognitive and moral dissonance going on that I was clearly not finding a balance.

After a significant love affair with my first male lover, I acquired herpes. At the same time, I started my first hospital job as an RN. I plunged into a depression that has claimed me off and on to this day. From that time on I blamed myself for all my sexual desires and felt guilty for every sexual affair after.

Looking back, it was a constant struggle to hone in on the kind of physical sexual intimate experience I desired in the deepest part of my being. It was an experience I was looking for to liberate my soul and my body and my mind.

My periods had always been regular. My mom was fertile. I was very afraid of becoming pregnant unplanned.

Wow. Writing those words actually makes me feel incredibly sad. I wish someone had given me a different message about that. I know from being a nurse the importance of being able to control our fertility. In my case, I wish someone had said, don't worry about it, you'll be fine if you get pregnant or not.

I dutifully took birth control. It did help with my moods. I liked missing periods sometimes. It made planning my sex life a lot more convenient. I did miss it a little but felt somewhere in the back of my head and from all the messages I was getting "you've got lots of time." I'll have access to my cycle again. No big deal. I understood my cycle pretty well, the crests and waves of mood, desire, body feelings. It was a rhythm I now weep and long for. I got a Mirena IUD because the pills and patches made me feel too weird. It was great—mindless birth control while I was in grad school! It was a less systemic hormone, less affect on my brain, and it didn't hurt. My period stopped. I was super happy.

Little did I know it was bridging me into menopause.

Looking back—yikes—the signs were there, subtle and sad, my body telling me what was happening. I wish I'd had the body wisdom to know the changes.

By age thirty-six, I was perimenopausal. I asked my dad the doctor about the skin changes I was having, knowing something was shifting. My ovulation was incredibly painful, more than ever. My sex drive ramped up like something I had never experienced.

I finished grad school for my ARNP and felt completely lost and burned out. Something had to change. I had a desperate feeling that something new and different needed to happen. I was ready to take some risks that were totally uncalculated and mine—really truly mine.

A close friend opted for single motherhood by choice with a donor. After some thought and "if I don't try I'll regret it" feelings, I proposed a queer family with my close gay friends. They were game. I asked for permission, or rather a blessing, from my family. They said, do it.

I had my IUD removed. I did queer family research. I tracked my cycle. Everyone congratulated me. I went on one desperate love affair after another looking for something. I hired a doula. And then, I had a really, really long period. Almost a month and a half. I called my doctor. We did a test. She said, I'm sorry, you are menopausal. I said, okay, how menopausal. She said, very.

I saw a fertility doctor who said I had a less than 1 percent chance of conceiving and that I had five follicles. Dad said, get sperm in there. We inseminated. Nothing happened. My periods stopped. My potential dads stopped talking to me. My friends said, you might recover. My mother said, we still love you. My sister-in-law said, I would have your baby. All my friends said, you can still be a mother. My body said, we're done.

My being said, WAIT. WHAT IS HAPPENING?!

I cried a lot for a long time. I thought about death. A lot. My maiden self rummaged around like a ghost. A mother baby self evaporated just as she was getting started, like Eurydice, pulled back out of my loving grasp. A crone self showed up and said, well, that's how it goes.

I felt stuck. I still feel stuck. I feel like a third gender, an old man, a strange lump, a silent clam on the bottom of the sea, the party chaperone who'd rather be at home, REALLY, REALLY LONELY.

Men said to me, menopause? What's that? I had yet to have a lover that understood what it meant. It was a drag to explain it. So I just referred to it as a "medical condition." I said that about two times and then I decided I was done having sex with anyone.

I tried yoni eggs, I tried baths, I tried acupuncture, I tried herbs, I tried counseling, I tried meditation, I tried dancing, I tried yoga, I tried Prozac. They all helped a little.

What really helped was tuning into my own body and tuning out all the Internet, people, advice, consolation, misunderstanding, etcetera, ETCETERA.

Not to say I didn't gather helpful information and support from all those things but none of them could tell me what my body didn't already know: IT WAS ALL OKAY AND AS IT SHOULD BE.

Today I had a conversation with my dad the doctor. He said he told someone about my condition and her response was "What a relief!" He said, I know you talk about all the bad things about it but you know, there might be some advantages too. I knew that, but a lot of me is still grieving at the same time that I am embracing the gifts, the really, really lovely gifts of menopause.

It's hard to celebrate alone. It's also hard to celebrate and grieve in public at the same time. People have a hard time with that. It's terribly awkward.

At the very least, menopause has taught me that. Grief and celebration happen in tandem, wisdom is in the body, community and womb wisdom is how you access those things.

Speak your truth, my new crone self says, it's the only way we can find ourselves and each other.

In retrospect:

I wish someone, society, some authority, some communal recognition could have been given to me to express the powerful things I was feeling and experiencing. It is worth likening to adolescence. It is a huge and immense transformation. Being a teenager feels easier than menopause. You have lots of adults (hopefully) and other teens that you get to be blissfully immersed with while you go through a transformation. Society holds you a little. There was no holding for me in menopause. It was fast and furious and full of denial. It was a cresting ravenousness for truth and feeling followed by a surrender and grief to letting go of all that appetite. It was all natural but made me feel so unnatural.

If I could have done it all over again, people would have stopped and sat with me for each hot flash to feel the radiating truths pushing out of my body. Each lover would have surrendered willing and trustfully to my aching desires, for there was genuine celebration of our connection and a frank desire for their uniqueness. Each person would have held my hand while my tears of grief poured out of me about all the loss and beauty and disappointment of my life.

When I was sitting in the fertility clinic waiting for my ultrasound to help determine my fertility, I saw my baby. I laid on the exam table asking whatever might hear me, my body, my destiny, my timeline: Would there be a family, a baby in my future? The answer was a vision of my baby—a boy, asking to be born—waiting for his blessing to come. It felt huge and precarious and real. I'm still mourning this unrealized life today. As I reflect back on my visions at that time for my life, it is now clear my body was at a burning decision point. I wish I'd had the womb wisdom to know the value of that pivot.

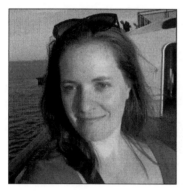

Meredith Kriebel is trained as a Doctor of Nursing Practice, Family Nurse Practitioner. She practices primary care embedded in outpatient mental health and in the homeless shelter system, all in the Seattle area. She is a daughter of the Olympic Peninsula on the Northwest Coast, born of love from two compassionate intelligent souls, a doctor and an artist. She is the sister of a great and wise man, for whom she lives in gratitude. She is an aunt to many powerful emerging beings shaped by this same beautiful place.

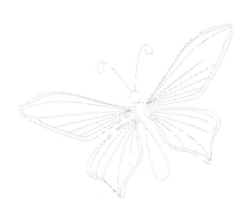

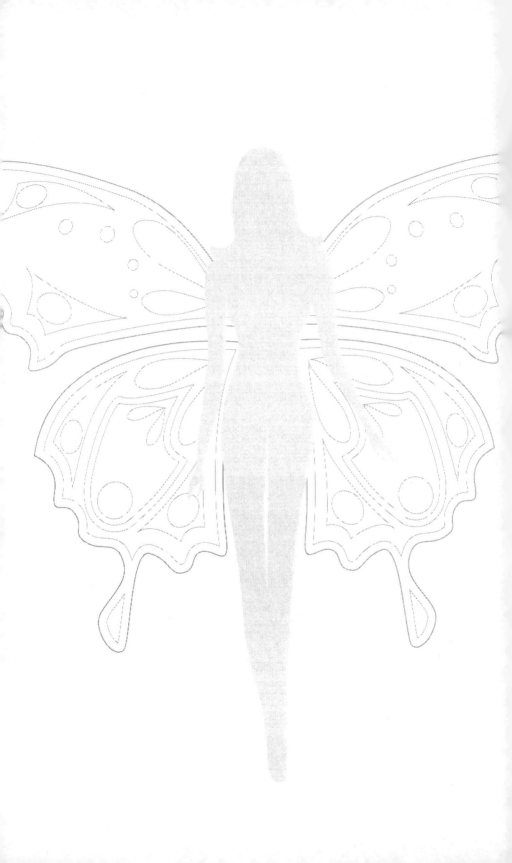

14

Embracing Change With Curiosity and Wonder

JUDY LENDSEY

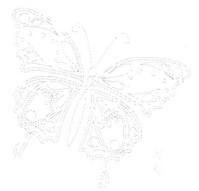

I was thirty-two when I was diagnosed with Stage 4 Non-Hodgkins Lymphoma. One day I was working full time and going to school full time, and the next day I was investigating clinical trials, pathology reports, and best possible prognosis options. People talked to me about getting "back to my old self" in no time at all, or how soon everything could be "back to normal," as if that were the goal. But it was clear to me relatively early on that everything was changing and there was no going "back" to anything. And so began my journey through change, and the first changes I became very aware of were the ones in my body and the way it functioned.

I tend to be a planner and live from a very organized place. I like things in their place, and I do best when I follow a scheduled routine. But I was about to take an abrupt turn I hadn't anticipated at all. I was on an aggressive form of chemotherapy. Almost immediately, I stopped menstruating. It was evident to me that the oncology team was approaching this as something that was not on our list of concerns at the moment. I felt as though there was a tradeoff being bargained, and my life was hanging in the balance. Yes, I was not having periods anymore, but their main goal was to get me in remission, and my uterus functionality—along with many other symptoms and results—was considered collateral damage.

I didn't get hot flashes or mood swings, at least not from per-imenopause or menopause symptoms. I did experience all the symptoms of actively going through chemotherapy, and that was not the most fun I've ever had in my life. Nothing felt the same. In fact, everything felt so different. I did my best to demonstrate that I wasn't changing. I'd go to all the places I could go that I usually went to, acted as close to "my normal self" as I could, and kept the appearance that this was temporary: I was going *through* it, and at some point I would not be going through it anymore, it would be behind me, in the past, and I could move on.

The thing about change of any kind—going through "the change" or having a life experience that changes you—is you don't go back: You move forward. You become more of the person you're supposed to be and, if you allow it, you grow into a bigger version of you that dreams, lives, and loves in a bigger way. I see people resisting change. If the interface on our computer looks different, we say, "I'm not used to it" or "it looks so different" and we discuss this with everyone we come in contact with that day. In actuality, everything is changing all the time—even ourselves. But we get so caught up in routines and being able to know before something happens so we feel comfortable and informed. We don't want to be taken off guard.

When I was done with chemotherapy, I wanted to learn about healthy people and how they did what they did and, more importantly, how I could do it. I looked at how I could recover from the massive amounts of medications that were pumped through my system and live close to a normal life. For me, this came back to diet and lifestyle. Thus I began another journey within this detour from corporate life to illness and back to wellness again.

Did you know that women in China don't go through menopause but for one week, and the sensation is similar to a stiff neck?

Why, I wondered, do women in China have such an easy transition my friends were suffering from hormonal disruption, hot flashes, facial hair, mood swings, and many more symptoms?

I believe it comes down to diet. Once I began to make changes to what I was eating, I began to menstruate again. I began to feel like a woman again; I felt alive again. My periods weren't regular and were nowhere near normal five to seven days of flow like I was used to, but I felt like something was happening, that my body was beginning to function again. That, to me, was a sure sign that I was doing something I should be doing and my body was recognizing it. Over time, and incorporating healthy changes into my daily routine, I began to notice more regularity in the months of ovulation and menstruation. I was really happy that these changes were taking place. I took them as a sign of moving in the right direction or having a positive effect on what was happening in my body and life.

I have more years healthy with the diet and lifestyle changes than I had in remission from chemotherapy, and I'm pretty pleased about that. I have followed a program that I put together for myself regarding my health, which is specifically designed for me, by me, all about me. I revise it when I learn new things. I'm always open to trying things and learning about how these changes can positively affect my main goal of being a healthy and happy person.

Now at forty-six and healthy, I am in the beginning stages of perimenopause or menopause symptoms. And I'm thankful. I am starting to have missed cycles and show the signs of being in menopause, which is so much better feeling than being thrown into it like I was during chemotherapy. I embrace change in all its forms and experience life the way I came here to experience it: alive and well.

No longer resisting change, I'm comfortable in my own body and my own life. And I'm helping other people to embrace the changes in their bodies and lives. I hope that for each of you—no matter how life has shown up for you in your experience—that you can find ways to observe what a situation is attempting to teach you. I learned a lot about myself through this whole experience, some of those things I liked very much and wanted to polish and refine, and other things I didn't care for and wanted to form new habits around. I am grateful now, for how it all came to be, because I don't believe I would have learned these things any other way.

I hope that you, too, can find the blessing in the life experiences that have shaped you into the person that you are today. Connect with others going through similar experiences or who need help getting from where they are to their next step can make all the difference. This process of "change" is easier when we do it together, feeling supported, being heard and understood. Who else can understand what we're going through better than other women with the same or similar feelings or experiences? I often remind myself of the progress I have made, and I assist other women who are in the process of change to do the same. Chart things for yourself and be very aware of the efforts you are making in taking great care of yourself. You will notice that this feels very good. And you know what happens when we do something that feels very good, don't you? We want to do it again and again. And we should!

I'm here cheering for you, hoping that you'll take the opportunity to face the changes in your life with curiosity and wonder, replacing dread and fear of the unknown with an openness to experience life and who you are becoming in a whole new way. It's an adventure. If you notice, when we get too comfortable, things change—and we adapt and move forward with a new outlook and a fresh feeling of amazement. Comfort zones don't cultivate growth. Staying the same isn't an option—not even if we wish it were. And so I invite you to embrace change, in all its mystery and unforeseeable essence, and to be open to what it wants to communicate through you.

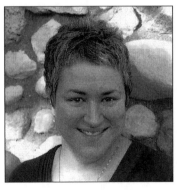

Judy Lendsey is a daughter, sister, friend, energy worker, coach, and a mentor who enjoys healthy relationships, healthy food, great music, great connections, learning new things, meeting new people, and helping people who are passionate about their health find ways to live their best lives. Her cancer experience changed her life in many ways. After conventional treatment, she found a way that worked better for her than the life she was living before cancer.

Learn more: *www.judylendsey.com*

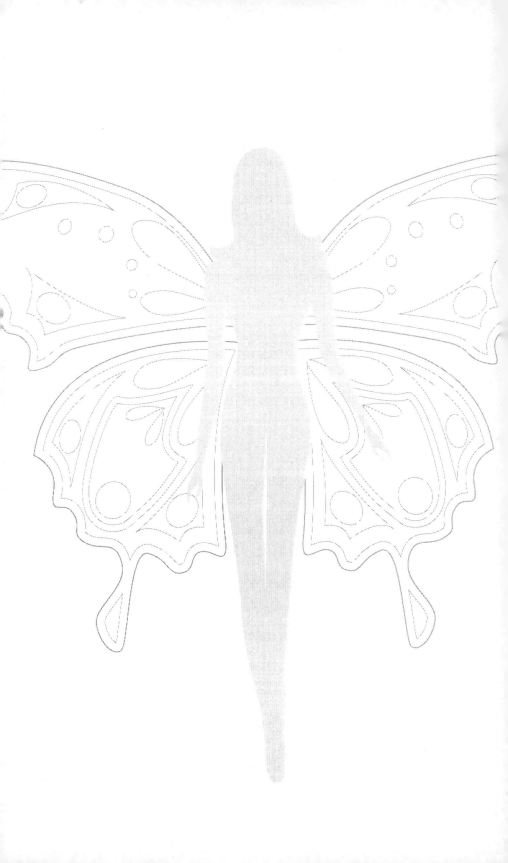

15

Cycles of Magic and Wisdom Highlights

DEBORAH LEEANN MORLEY

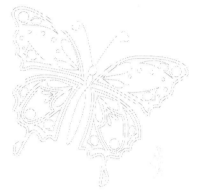

I've been called "Magic Lady," for my resourcefulness and ability to create something from nothing. Most of my life, I was seen as someone who could fall into a pile of s**t and come out smelling like roses. My mostly charmed life has been full of wonderful experiences and people serendipitously crossing my path. My story of falling in love and marrying sounds like a fairy tale, and our first year of marriage was spent traveling on my new husband's sabbatical and living in three gorgeous cities, all beginning with S, and which happen to have stunning harbors—Stockholm, Sydney, and San Francisco. However, the magical experiences I created were always for others. I hadn't yet learned how to create magic for my Self. To get there, I took a circuitous journey from premenopause through perimenopause to postmenopause.

PREMENOPAUSE

Twenty years ago, we were visiting friends on Maui and my husband wanted to visit a local nude beach. Normally, this would have totally freaked me out. Sharing my body with the world? What about all those young, beautiful, toned, tanned show-offs?

This time was different, though. I was 7½ months pregnant! I was in love with my body, its shape, and the miracle blooming within. My hormones were amazingly balanced, my hair and skin gorgeous. I was happy, excited, and loving sex—ready to play at the beach in all of my natural goddess glory! The saltwater was warm yet refreshing and I floated with the extra buoyancy of my belly. This new version of skinny-dipping was pure blissful freedom and still a vivid memory for me. *All* of Me felt enveloped, caressed, and gently supported.

There was a beautiful Nordic-looking couple next to us with amazing sculpted muscles and curves. Intrigued, I couldn't keep my eyes off of them. My gaze was not one of jealousy—which might have been my reaction at another time—but one of curiosity and appreciation of the gorgeous human form. Instead of being self-conscious, I felt sexy as I sensually strutted my belly and I to and from my towel—feeling others' eyes watching me. Such a relief to not feel the need to hold in my stomach!

When the Beautiful Man—who was, and still is, the most well-endowed male human I've personally encountered—got up to follow me into the water, I felt a rush of attraction, desire, and wonder that maybe he found my maternity status sensual as well. In the water, with my eyes closed and fantasizing, I sensed his nearness and all kinds of crazy images played across my mind. As I opened my eyes, Beautiful Woman was coming into the water as well. Her breasts so perfect, her buttocks so toned, she knew she was the envy of all women on the beach that day.

I went back to my musings and lusty play within and swam out farther into the playful waves. This magical and miraculous body and I were one, gloriously, giddily happy in love with living.

My hair was still dark and natural then, at thirty-eight, not one gray hair in sight.

PERIMENOPAUSE

In another five years, I was entering perimenopause. At forty-two? Really? Two quick pregnancies after that first—one not fulfilled—and a year after delivery of our second darling daughter, I started the intense and crazy periods. I went back on the pill. I tried natural hormones. I felt cranky, irritable, and tired all the time. I felt that the parenting of two small ones was almost too big of a task for someone as old as me. I began to hate having sex. My hair started thinning. My adrenals were shot. Hot flashes were frequent, and they were awkwardly difficult to explain to my friends who were not at the same place on their women's journey. The arguments between my husband and I escalated as I cut my hair shorter. I was getting the first few strands of silver in my beautiful dark hair.

In another five years, my periods were over but the other symptoms were still present. My weight was not budging even though we walked everywhere while living in Australia without a car. I cooked most meals with healthy and natural ingredients. I was studying naturopathic regimens. And yet I was unable to sustain the joy and freedom of living in such a naturally stunning resort town. My marriage was falling apart.

Magic was all around me—in the nature preserve behind our building, on the 270-degree horizon as I witnessed the sun and moon rising, in the ocean that I walked by daily on my way to and from town taking kids to school or carrying groceries, and in the shining happy faces of people playing at the beaches on vacation. Where was mine?

POSTMENOPAUSE

Three years later, we were separated and back in the States. I managed to find a perfect smaller home in the same neighborhood as my husband so the kids could still walk to and from school, their friends' houses, and between their our houses. My magic began to return. I intuitively moved from medical to full alternative care. My hot flashes diminished noticeably, my weight dropped, my joy increased, and I slept all night. I began to masturbate several times a week, as my sex drive returned… oh, the joy of my body! It was like we were reunited in a love affair!

The alimony was only for one year, and it took another year to get clear on who I was, what I wanted to do, and which organizations I wanted to serve. I found myself drawn to feminine principles, spirituality, and ways of being. I received Feminine Leadership coaching and learned how to integrate my passion for Native American teachings, the Mother Earth care regimen I lived by, my health coach training, and previous management consulting experience. All was folded into who I was becoming. Each step and lesson was like a stepping stone on the divine path back to Me.

Like a Warrior Priestess, I packed my medicine bag and let my Intuition guide me. Networking and professional development led me to the right people and to the most desirable projects with two highly regarded organizations in the nonprofit arena. The work was easy for me, providing part-time income while I gained as much credibility in the nonprofit community as I had in my previous consulting experience in the corporate world. I began to see that I could *create* for myself and allow that to *be*. I could receive these gifts in a way that was new to me.

At the same time, I had called in a sex and spiritual partner, and when we met, I was amazed at my accuracy in manifesting! He was exactly that, though emotionally not available to me at that time. This served me well, as I wasn't ready to dive in deeply, either. During our time together, he has taught me so much but mostly allowed me to grow and embrace a new form of self-love and acceptance. He lets me cry and rant and be crazy angry—all new forms of self-expression for me. Now that I know I don't scare him when I act out, that part of me rarely needs to do it. He taught me to sing, too, which helped me find my "voice" for which I will always be grateful. It had been squelched as a child when I heard "Children are to be seen, not heard," and was also told to "Mouth the words, honey. You can't sing."

I can now see my Self as he does (and maybe most others, too) as beautiful—inside and out. I can look adoringly at my body, love the wrinkles, cellulite, and belly. It's such a source of joy! I *am* the full spectrum from strong and independent to needy and childish. And, the best part? He doesn't run away. And that gives me permission to love and tenderly accept those shadow parts of me that just need to be seen and loved. We continue to redefine "relationship" with our day-by-day appreciation for what we have in each other—best friends who *see* each other and support and hold each other's dreams to co-create them together or singularly. His Magic feeds my Magic in a synergistic way—a beautiful blending of the Divine Masculine and Divine Feminine.

It's now been a decade since my periods have ended, and I'm calling my silver highlights near my temples and in my bangs my *Wisdom* highlights. A young person told me that I had earned them and should not cover them with color but display them proudly. Now those are full-circle, words of wisdom—from a maiden to a vivacious crone like myself.

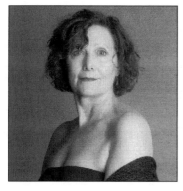

Deborah LeeAnn Morley is a women's leadership catalyst and teacher of the Art of Feminine Presence™. She has made contributions to both corporate and nonprofit worlds for more than thirty years as an organizational development consultant and human resources professional. Deborah melds her passions for community building, health/wellness, and women's studies, resulting in resourceful and intuitive leadership development coaching programs and trainings for powerful and feminine women. From workaholic to stay-at-home mom to divorced entrepreneur raising two teenage daughters, Deborah is an avid fan of nature, hiking, health/wellness rituals, organic gardening, and finding art in the everyday.

Learn more: www.deborahleeann.com

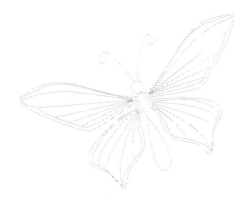

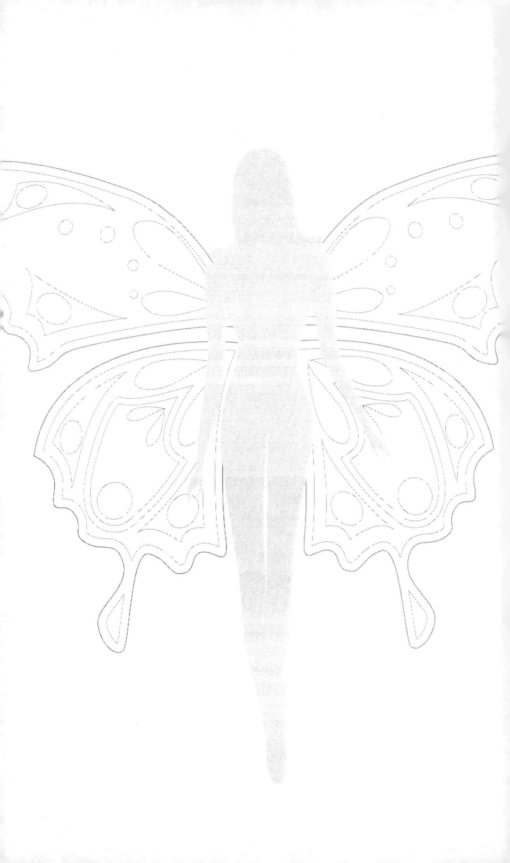

16

A Prescription for Exercise

MARIE MOZZI

Just as no two women are alike, no two women experience this menopause journey quite the same way. As a result, relief of symptoms varies from woman to woman, making any universal "prescription" ineffective. We blame those "crazy hormones," and we believe we have no control over the process. But there *is* one thing that can alleviate or reduce menopausal symptoms: exercise. Research definitely supports the exercise helps.

Exercise is a universal answer to so many health-related issues, so why would menopause be different? When exercise is a part of the equation, the changes that can result from movement come from the acute results, not the piece of trying to attempt to "correct" the hormonal changes. Oh they're coming, they're there, or they are in place. But exercise will ease the blow.

Research demonstrates that exercise is a key piece in dealing with the multitude of symptoms that affect any women going through the menopausal journey. The benefits range from decreased anxiety and depression to enhanced feelings of wellness. The fatigue and muscle pain that can be associated with menopause can be minimized with exercise. Quality and length of sleep can be improved with exercise as well. Lower cholesterol, better blood sugar control, better weight control, and stronger bones are the gifts of exercise.

The three components of exercise that need to be incorporated for overall health are the same for peri- and postmenopausal women as for everyone else: cardiovascular fitness, strength training, and flexibility/balance. Each component is necessary to create a truly functional and strong body, inside and out.

Cardiovascular exercise is about getting your heart rate up into a training zone, one that challenges your heart and you lungs. Elevate your heart rate and reap the benefits immediately. The recommendation for cardio is thirty minutes, five times a week. Even cumulative workouts count, which means that even ten minutes throughout the day releases endorphins and promotes an overall sense of well-being.

Resistance training is the next key component in a successful exercise program. Whether you use bands, weighted balls, ropes, tubes, or simply your own body weight, the options are endless. The most important piece is to consistently increase weight over time. Muscle endurance is important to "prep" and build overall support in the muscle. The next step is strength. If the weight gets too easy, don't be afraid to lift a bit more. Strength gains are being made, and that's the way muscle is developed. Muscle is what burns fat at rest and helps get rid of tricky areas like the belly.

Visceral fat, better known as belly fat, can lead to many aggravating symptoms associated with menopause. The increase in body fat usually occurs during and after menopause, which shows up in symptoms like hot flashes, night sweats, interrupted sleep, mood swings, and poor self esteem. As belly fat increases, so does insulin resistance, which means we crave more simple carbohydrates in the form of sweets and sugar.

Start by getting a full-body workout incorporating favorite resistance tools. Working more than one muscle at a time—using the body as a whole—burns more calories.

Resistance training should be done at least three times a week. If you're not sure what to do, consider hiring a qualified trainer so that you can be effective and efficient with your workouts.

Finally, integrate into your exercise program moves or workouts that encourage flexibility and relaxation. Yoga is a perfect example as it focuses on slow deliberate postures that incorporate the breath. Work on flexibility and continue to elongate muscles that ensure you have "flexible strength." This prevents injury and promotes that mind-body connection.

Move, dance, and express yourself. Your cardio workouts should be more than walking on a treadmill or riding a stationary bike: Instead, move in a variety of planes and giving the body a sense of freedom and expression. Find an activity that moves you right and left, up and down, forward and backward.

One concept often neglected in "exercise programs" is the benefit of movement and the flow of energy it creates. The energy centers in the body are connected to major organ or glands. Each of these energy centers are referred to as *chakras*. Without getting too technical, I'll tell you that chakras can create a spinning vortex of energy and create a vacuum in the center that can draw anything to it on a vibrational level. For many women, these chakras are stuck, or blocked, and energy doesn't flow at all. The second chakra is located below the navel and is the color orange. It is responsible for creativity and feelings. That is why I am such an advocate of movement in your exercise program that generates your body moving up, down, right, left and, forward, and back. Dance, rocking of the hips, and freedom of movement in which self-expression exists is so vitally important for women at any stage of the health game. Emotions are housed, stuck, and hidden in the area of hips and illiospoas, tucked far away. Moving those hips creates some energy and opportunity to move with freedom and self-expression. The release of blocked energy and emotions may be subtle, but it alone is empowering and freeing.

The saying "dance like nobody is watching" has some merit. Menopause is a time to release, stimulate energy, and encourage creativity while finding energy in the freedom of just letting go. Abort the treadmill and the elliptical trainer for a bit, and learn to move with a sense of freedom. Take a dance class, move to music at home, and or find a trainer that will get you moving in all directions.

Do what is fun. Grab a partner or exercise with a group of women. Whatever will add to your success is what getting through this transitional chapter of life is what this is all about!

This process of changing hormone levels can last for more than a decade. Don't wait to start exercising. We *know* that exercise benefits the body in hundreds of ways, and we have been told this by every health professional everywhere. But it is human nature to wait until we are confronted with a life-changing event that screams, "Do it!" Menopause *is* that event. Do it!

Though it's never too late to start an exercise program, sooner is better than later. If you are in the throes of hot flashes and hormonal body disputes on a daily basis, get on it! It is more difficult to start a program when the body is going through hormonal fluctuations resulting in a variety of physiological and psychological changes. Natural body changes are occurring, no matter what. The key is to remember exercise will bring an overall body health that will help support the body as a whole. Choose activities that you enjoy so you will comply with making this a part of your life. This is not a short-term fix but a path to sustaining your involvement. With that in mind, create an exercise program with conviction, purpose, and intention.

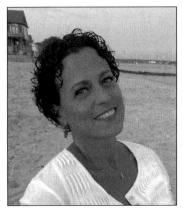

Marie Mozzi is a vitality coach with a passion for motivating others to live their authentic life by finding balance between movement, food, and real-life issues. She is a fitness and wellness professional with more than twenty years of experience and holds numerous certifications and awards in the Spa and Fitness arenas. Marie creates success for companies and individuals by integrating the mind, body, and spirit connection into her programs. Marie consults, presents, and motivates audiences of all ages throughout the United States and lives what she teaches. Her favorite project is being a mom!

Learn more: www.GetRealWithMarie.com

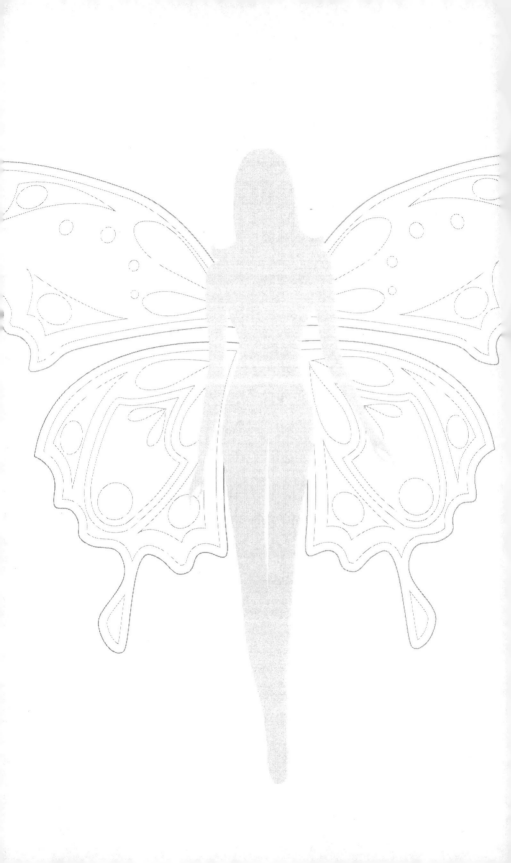

The Masquerade Is Over: Shedding Masks at Midlife

DR. SIRENA PELLAROLO

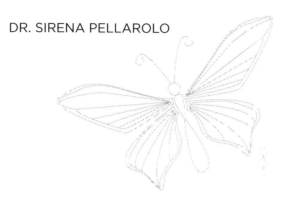

The room is dimly lit by candles on an altar. Journals, photos, and rose petals are scattered on the floor. Incense is burning, and meditative music plays in the background. Participants take seats on the floor, a womblike structure of silk cloth overhead, flanks the semicircle. Two fairy-like ushers welcome the participants and gift each one of them with a candle. My daughters Paloma and Violeta go around the circle lighting candles. Then Violeta turns around the water stick, signaling the beginning of the ceremony.

Paloma stands by the mouth of the fabric womb and reads a bilingual poem about birthing and lighting, "Alumbramiento": "The maidens bring candles and multicolored fires to light the descent. They are the ones (. . .) who find the magic of widening my hips and give way to the unstoppable irruption of silence. It is time to rejoice!"

I emerge from the womb dressed in white. My daughters hold my hands, help me rise, and anoint me. One of the ushers illumines the birth scene with a candle.

Women form a semicircle around me. In the middle of the circle I proudly introduce my new identity. Spreading out my arms I say, "I am Sirena Próspera del Mar, *hija de la Luna, curandera y ñusta, adoradora de Iemanja.*"

And I add,

I accept my newness. I discard the old, the useless. Just as I cut the withering leaves of my favorite plant to allow the vital energy to grow new shoots, I solemnly proclaim today that I am shedding old masks, belief systems, habits, and behaviors that are withering my soul. I release fear and guilt. I let go of insecurities and feelings of unworthiness. I discard any sense of lack, resentfulness, or frustration. I discard impatience, mistrust, and the need for external validation. I transform what I shed into love, compassion, wholeness, confidence, and bountiful abundance. I stand tall in my truth knowing that I am a radiant Sirena wading through the seaweed, in service to the most high.

This public rite of passage of rebirthing myself at midlife aided by my daughters and witnessed by some of my fellow journey travelers was the final project of a Science of Mind class I was taking at the (then) Agape Church of Religious Science in December 2000. The ceremony had been inspired by a powerfully transformative dream I had had a month before where I witnessed myself lying on the floor of one of our classes, legs spread out, giving birth. As the birth progressed, I noticed the head of a fully grown woman emerging from my body: the face of the newborn was my own; I was birthing myself. That was indeed a very graphic way my subconscious mind had of communicating how I was literally—rather physically—embodying my own rebirth! I was forty-five then and entering perimenopause, a time in my life (and the life of so many other women) of intense transformation, typically marked by the crumbling and disintegrating of accepted structures and belief systems. It was time to shed the masks!

As we enter midlife, with the rebalancing of our hormonal system, we women are immersed in an alchemic process of purification by fire, whereby anything that doesn't serve us anymore melts away. In this process of distillation, we let go of the social masks that we had been wearing until then—the mother, the professional woman, the daughter, the aunt—all those roles that used to define us while we were taking care of others or pursuing our own careers. Meno-pause demands of us to look at those masks and decide whether they still serve us. If we dare to shed the ones that are no longer useful and plunge courageously into the cauldron of transformation, we are brought back home to the essence of who we really were even before our childbearing years.

In my own life experience, there was still much more pain and dragons to slay, but my heroine's journey was well under way, deep and intentional. The path had been drawn by the enactment of my rebirth ushered by my daughters, my midlife midwives. They were showing me the way toward what I was being called to become as I traversed this portal of menopause: a midlife midwife, accompa-nying other women in their own rebirthing journeys, a process that requires all the support we can receive from our sisters.

The transformation had started earlier that year, exactly on the eve of my forty-fifth birthday. It was the first night of a women's retreat, during a time when I was undergoing a quantum shift in consciousness. In my journals I kept record of the intense psychic upheaval that punctuated the adoption of a new identity through images, dreams, and longings. I also took pains to note that this particular event was allowed to emerge during a powerful premen-strual time that would peak in the shedding of blood on full moon. No accident here, as Dr. Northrup reminds us, because the increased levels of progesterone during PMS activate "the more intuitive parts of our brain" making "the veil between our conscious and uncon-scious selves (…) thinner (…) as we prepare to give birth to nothing less than ourselves."

I clearly knew that it was a time to change gears as many areas in my life had become unviable and my whole energetic field was desperately yearning to spin into a new version of myself. Hence my prayers that night to receive in dreams the true way of naming me by my forty-fifth birthday. Notations in my journal give account of the realization that my new identity was related to water and the oceanic goddess Iemanja. That night I dreamt very clearly the name "Sirena" handwritten in pencil on a piece of paper. This shocking revelation of a name that seemed quite extraneous then took me to a frantic search for meaning of what this new identity was asking me to become.

The conscious diving into the aquatic medium of emotions and corporeal awareness reminiscent of my intrauterine life was clearly rendering my intellectual academic persona obsolete. As a college professor and a single mom, I had chosen to favor rational faculties that supported myself and my family. This utilitarian approach was at the expense of the development of my fiery imagination and the stirrings to move forward by the power of the heart. Things needed to change now. The submerging into an amniotic environment of dreamlike pulsations unearthed a buried personal mythology that had the potential to requalify Dr. Pellarolo's structured persona.

It's been exactly fourteen years since that flash of intuition put me in touch with my core essence. Today I'm writing about the shedding of masks at midlife on Winter Solstice: the darkest and longest night of the year that gives birth to the Light Child, the ushering of the new. What an appropriate time to talk about another rebirthing as I cross one more threshold toward elderhood! I am fully retired now, an experience I've been yearning for decades. I am excited and scared. I will turn sixty next June. I feel I'm on the brink of entering another transformative portal, similar to the one I entered at forty-five. Reflecting on those years will hopefully illumine the path I'm starting to tread now.

However, I feel there are still some loose ends that need to be brought together. I realize now that I have never fully embodied the greatness of la Sirena. The process has remained slightly in stasis, in Nepantla, that liminal space in between, a threshold that I did not dare to cross completely due to my hesitancy to face the emergence of my magnificent self. Interestingly, as I am in the process of making sense of the origins of my midlife transformation, my body is reacting with a vengeance to this paralysis and is pushing me to look at what still needs attention. I have developed an extreme case of eczema on my face that surrounds my mouth and my left eye. I have tried everything possible to heal it, and it's still there. I would like to think that the rawness of my skin indicates that I'm still shedding old masks, those that had become stuck to my countenance as I held firmly to old identities.

I renounce everything—even those obstinate masks—to have it all. That is why I have decided to take a radical stance and let go of 90 percent of my humble belongings, those that are still imbued with the clingy energy of fear and insecurity. This shedding will allow the new to completely emerge and integrate the disparate aspects of my psyche. I am also leaving the city that I have called home for the past twenty-six years. The stripping of old identities will hopefully open me up to grant conscious permission to La Sirena to finally come forth in her splendid brilliance. Masks gone, the truth of whom I really am shining forth. No more struggling, no more obligations. I finally claim my simple and authentic self. No posturing, no masks. The masquerade is finally over. *Vamos a andar…*

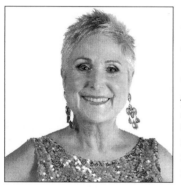

Sirena Pellarolo, Ph.D., your Midlife Midwife, is an international author, speaker and holistic healer. She supports women in their menopause years to recover their juiciness and dive full on into a vibrantly healthy and fulfilled second half of their lives. With thirty years experience in self development, health and wellness, Sirena believes in a holistic and empowered approach to traverse the portal of menopause through self-awareness, emotional, mental, and physical detoxing.

Her bilingual programs inspire individuals to reconnect with their bodies, minds and spirits by going back to the basics of a healthy lifestyle: a personalized nutrient-rich diet, energizing physical movement and a meaningful spiritual practice.

A board-certified holistic health coach, raw food educator, detox expert, radio host and blogger, Sirena is Professor Emerita of Spanish and Latin American Cultural Studies. She has authored and published numerous articles and two books on Latin American performance and gender studies, globalization and new social movements. Sirena is a compelling public speaker offering wellness seminars in English and Spanish. Her forthcoming book Recover Your Juiciness: A 30-Day DIY Guide for an Empowered and Healthy Menopause *will be published next fall by Flower of Life Press.*

*Learn more: **www.SirenaPellarolo.com***
*Email: **info@sirenapellarolo.com***

18

Yoga + Breast Cancer = Extraordinary Compassionate Body

FELICIA LANE SAVAGE

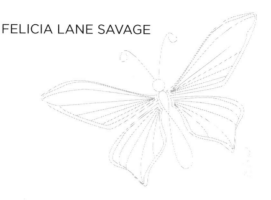

It was a Friday in April 2009. I remember because Maya and I were staying with my parents, and Cleveland was in Minneapolis going to graduate school for Mechanical Engineering. We were in transition from one apartment to another. I was hoping to fall in love with Mr. HotLanta and move there, but my knight decided to ride his steed into the sunset without me on it. So, in walks Cancer. Breast Cancer came bursting into my life like an unannounced old boyfriend at your wedding to the man of my dreams! Bam! Actually that is an extremely tall tale, I knew *something* was going on. I faintly remember a dream that showed me something with light was growing inside of me.

The phone call was my dearest Dr. Woodyear. She sounded like she had been perhaps crying as she managed to get out the words: I had Breast Cancer Stage 0.

"Well," I said, cool beans it is all right but I needed her advice as if I was her daughter or mother. What would she suggest?

She referred me to UPMC Shadyside Surgeon Dr. Smooth Chocolate Songbird Steven Evans. I decided that I wanted the cancer out by order of a lumpectomy, yesterday. The soonest they could schedule it was over Memorial Day weekend. Oddly, I felt great, physically—energetic and at the top of my YogaDiva-ness.

Maya didn't take the news too well. Cleveland seemed accepting; I was all right at the moment, and he was in the thick of school. I didn't feel pressed to say goodbye to anyone yet, so I took it in stride. After my surgery, my mom and dad sent Maya to Nashville for several weeks for a scholars program. I could focus on my self-awareness and self-care just like I had encouraged so many community members.

You see, my yoga practice is the standard by which I measure my life. Yoga is my refuge and go-to friend that has always supported me. To me, yoga and God are synonymous.

By then, I had practiced yoga for sixteen years and taught for a decade. I was working full time as a Health Coach/Yoga Instructor-Trainer for The Healthy Black Family Project, a successful collaboration between the University of Pittsburgh's Graduate School of Public Health-Center for Minority Health and many community organizations. The program provided access to BodyToning, yoga, water aerobics, African dance, nutrition class, chronic disease management, and cancer education to the predominantly Black population in the East Liberty/Larimer neighborhoods of the City of Pittsburgh. The project's goal was to assist community members to decrease the incidences of diabetes, cardiovascular disease, and hypertension in the targeted population.

I was the yoga instructor, and I had a disease. And so I decided that I would share my adventure with my students. When I went for a biopsy, the nurses were surprised that I didn't feel anything. I told them that I was in Jamaica on the beach eating mangoes and jackfruit, running on the beach and getting brown like a sweet cherry. I performed my breathing techniques that I have practiced for years, determined to enjoy each moment.

The biopsy proved to remove all of the cancer cells. When Dr. Evans performed the full lumpectomy, the pathology report came back clean! I remember right before the surgery the anesthesiologist and I had words about my nose ring. I didn't want to take it out; he insisted because of metal burns. That convinced me.

The surgery was successful. Dr. Evans said that I needed to take a two-week break from teaching and taking yoga classes. Several years earlier, I had started to train some of my students who showed themselves to be disciplined in their practice. Maya stepped up to lead classes.

After the surgery I began to take an estrogen blocker called Tamoxifen. It stopped my menses and made me so sleepy that I had to take a nap every day. I couldn't nap during my workday, so I stopped taking the prescription drug. Instead, I took WomenSense EstroSense, a dietary supplement with Indole-3 Carbinol and several herbs, that supports healthy balance of hormones, healthy breasts, effortless periods, and healthy PMS symptoms.

My PMS symptoms had been intense: fatigue, allergies, sleep disturbances, pajama-soaking night sweats, hot flashes during the day, mood swings, 25-pound weight gain, and quick-to-come-upon-me-irritability.

I was determined to take it all in stride, but I must admit the most annoying was me not having a flat belly anymore. I decided to love my more voluptuous body. For the first time in my life I understood what women had shared with me over the years: they had additional weight that they found it hard to get rid of. Empathy kicked in! I instantly understood how they felt. I felt ashamed that I really didn't understand even though I oftentimes felt I truly did understand. I was developing my Compassionate Body.

I continued to practice gentle yoga seven times a week, line dance at least once a week, taking the stairs, and eating a more conscious diet of mostly vegetarian with some fish and chicken. I had been a vegan for twelve years and pure vegetarian for six additional years. I gave up my vegetarian badge because I wanted to eat dairy occasionally and fish and chicken frequently, and I realized that I had been a self-righteous vegan and vegetarian! I might as well go and eat meat and not look down on others who make different decisions about their diet. Our diet doesn't bring us closer to God. If anything, our self-righteousness takes us further from the spirit of love.

My twenty-five-year-old practice continues to be one of being totally present in my body, being in tune with every ache, pain, and pleasure. I practice aromatherapy with essential oils: frankincense and peppermint to uplift me, and lavender and lemon to soothe my soul. I perform self-Reiki at the first sign of distress, placing my hands on my body wherever I feel to honor the moment. I frequently take body scans to just check-in with myself, because I really enjoy being alone with me. Most of the time, I am not lonely. But when I am, if I am feeling anxious I curl up into a side-lying child's pose with blankets, pillows, and bolsters surrounding me and I take myself to that safe, warm cocoon that feels of cashmere softness enveloping me with the Lord's most Blessed Assurance. Agape love.

I continue my practice of assisting community members in attaining their health and wellness goals through my yoga work. My students saw me go through thirty sessions of radiation with high-heeled shoes on for thirty days. Throughout that process, I shared that today was the rest of my life and I intended to celebrate every F$%^&*@ glorious moment.

My students saw me tired and drained and still going through my adventure with as much spice as I could muster up. They saw me weak in my left arm—and then gradually rebuilding strength over the next year, though never to its pre-cancer strength. They saw me buy new clothes that were larger than I have ever wore before and still prance around as the Queen of YogaDivaness that I am because I am here.

Through my meditation and stillness practice, I thank the Lord every day that I am here to celebrate with you all the sweet deliciousness of taking a breath of cold and frigid Pittsburgh air. I am full of thanks that I was blessed with a grateful spirit to navigate all of life's adventures with finesse and effortless effort just like the transition from warrior two to high lunge.

Let's slowly helicopter down to rest for a moment to sip the delectable moment of enjoying the present moment.

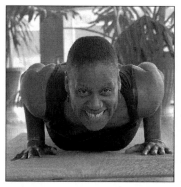

Felicia Lane Savage (MEd, 500 RYT) *is an exuberant African-American yogini. She has practiced Raja yoga for over twenty-five years and has taught for nineteen. Her practice influences her style of living, which is gratefully and joyfully integrated with friends and students from various backgrounds challenging her personal prejudices and biases, line dancing, gentle yoga, Reiki, contemplative self-awareness and self-care practices, conscientious eating practices that balance nutrition with deliciously diverse ethnic foods, and engaging, educating, and empowering others to live a healthier and happier existence in harmony with each other. She has enjoyed growing two adults: Cleveland, The Real Rocket Man, and Maya, The Fashionista Yogini Teacher.*

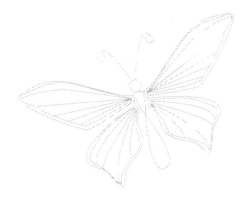

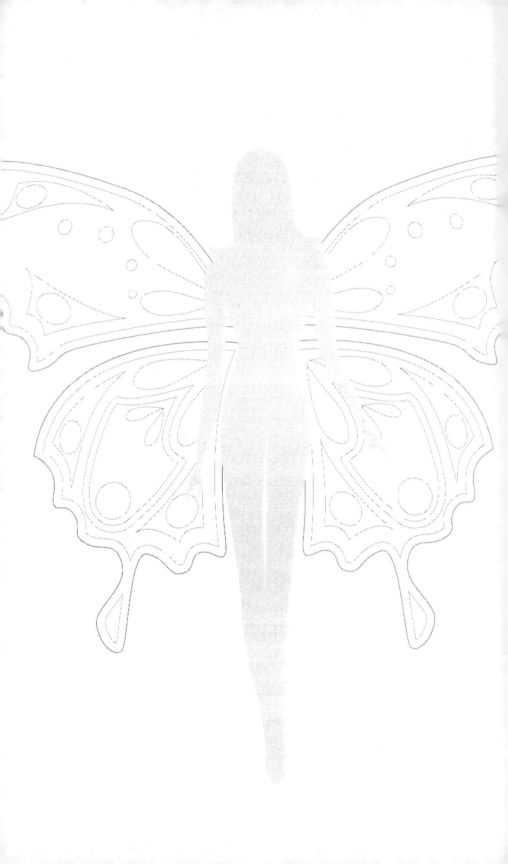

19

Wisdom of Weeds

MISCHA SCHULER

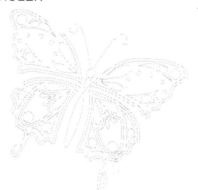

"I don't know what the hell you did, girl," Paula says. She sits up from the fluffy down blankets I had placed on the floor as a make-shift massage table. "But I can move my shoulder."

Paula, a phenomenal yoga teacher and Southern belle with a wicked wit, had offered herself as a human guinea pig. She and I are both of the same mind that the physical body can accumulate negative emotional experiences in weakened areas, causing pain or discomfort. I was in the process of learning shamanic techniques through a yearlong apprenticeship with a beloved mentor. Paula had presented with: "Menopause fucking sucks. What can you do for me?"

As a beginner, naturally my response was "I don't know" and then, "I've just learned an extraction technique. Let's see if that might make a difference for you."

Paula enthusiastically agreed to my removing any unnecessary "crap" that was no longer serving her Highest Good. To do this, I called in my guides, rattling and whistling in the four directions to bring myself into a trance-like state, and sprinkled salt water around us to clear us and summon us both to be present. I invited my extraction guide, a beautiful bird, to merge with my own energy field. Then, I sat, with bowl of water and dry towel, prepared to withdraw whatever I saw through my bird's eyes that didn't look appropriate in Paula's field.

What I "see" is color, and sometimes stuff—keys, baby carriages, dumbbells—in dark shades. Only if an item appears red or gold am I meant to mention it as something potentially significant. I draw out these items, which are sometimes two feet away from the body and other times require an "incision" to discard them. These items are separated from the energy field by my bird's wing tips and dropped into my bowl of water. I then dry my hands on the towel and continue the process until it feels complete. Then comes the process of rattling, singing, and toning to seal the energy body so that no other unwanted spirit power squeezes into the space.

"I didn't tell you about how my shoulder has been frozen since a disagreement I had with a friend a few years ago," Paula says. For the next two days, she emails and texts her astonishment and joy at comfortably engaging in yoga poses that she thought she'd never be able to do again in her life.

Before each shamanic session, I check in with my spirit guides to ask how they can help the person who is coming to see me. Often, I see in my mind's eye a brief story unfold, and this is something I am able to share with my client during our session together. Generally, I haven't met the people with whom I will be working in advance, and the vignettes I share provide an opening into discussing whatever topic might be bringing them to shamanism.

During a check-in before a visit with a woman in her mid-forties, I saw one of my animal guides fly toward me carrying a pink ribbon and received news that she would be experiencing a soul retrieval. A soul retrieval returns a part of a person's soul which has split away during a trauma. A trauma could be a car accident, loss of a loved one, surgery, shock, anything that causes a person to feel deep fear and a need to hide to feel safe. I told this client that she would be receiving a lost soul part and that I had seen a pink ribbon.

It wasn't until the end of the session when I described what I saw during her soul retrieval journey—that the pink ribbon had turned white and was returning to her as a symbol of acceptance—that she shared with me the missing puzzle piece. She was a breast cancer survivor and was currently working on bringing acceptance to her healing.

There are times, after the conclusion of extraction work, when a plant will come through to fill in the energetic space as I am working. This plant spirit comes in as a guide and healing ally for whomever is seeking support.

A woman at the end of her menopause came to see me with a vision concern. At the end of her extraction session, the plant Rue asked to be given to her as a guide. To invite the plant into her energetic field, I was asked to blow the plant spirit into both the woman's heart chakra and crown chakra. Now, this is a plant I don't know very well. I have grown it in my garden over a number of years, yet have never harvested it for herbal medicine. It is a powerful plant that has historically been used as an eye wash and has been associated with witches.

This woman, I learned as I journeyed for her, was given the gift of this vision challenge to support her in awakening her own inner intuitive vision. To inspire her to actively continue down this new path, to both heal her eyesight and to trust her inner wisdom, Rue came forth. I had this herb on hand in the form of a flower essence, and I sent her home with a bottle of the flower essence to take in drop doses (three drops, three times per day), to encourage her connection with her new plant guide. She can now call upon Rue for support when she is actively working on her intuitive receptivity.

My relationship with the plants grew out of a science background. I had a remarkable high school teacher during senior year, and I knew then that I wanted to teach young people about our relationship to the natural world. I earned a master's degree in the education field and quickly became disenchanted with teaching about our world within four walls. While a staff naturalist at an outdoor school, I discovered the herbal medicine curriculum at a local university. I knew of edible plants, and had been exploring that for some time, but plants as medicine? It was mind blowing.

Our master's-level program was rigorous and demanding and focused on physiology. Our teachers had great hearts and love for the plants, and there wasn't always space to hold the more subtle spiritual qualities that nature provides.

It was outside and after school that I began apprenticing with mentors and the plants themselves. With time I was able to trust and embrace the aspects of plant medicine that fall beyond the bounds of our cultural understanding. This is an evolution that has been and continues to be very personal.

One of the first plants to communicate with me (out of the blue) is Wild Carrot, *Daucus carota,* also known as Queen Anne's Lace. I was sitting in an herbal conference, wearing a name tag that, in addition to my own name, included the name Wild Carrot below it. Each woman at this conference was wearing a name tag with a plant. It was meant as a clever ice breaker; the goal was to find the other nine women who were wearing a name tag labeled with the same plant as one's own.

I didn't find my other women companions, but Wild Carrot did find me!

At some point, in the midst of a lecture, I looked down at my name tag, not knowing a damn thing about Wild Carrot; knew in an instant that the name of my future herbal practice would be Wild Carrot Herbs; and broke into silent tears. Of course, I wondered what the hell was going on with me and I quietly departed the talk to catch some air and found myself walking through the area of teachers' items and books for sale.

One booklet caught my attention. *Wild Carrot: A Plant for Conscious, Natural Contraception.*

This amazing plant is used to improve thyroid conditions as well as to support conception and contraception; these actions are dose- and timing-dependent. When taken daily, in the morning, much as it would be taken to support thyroid levels, it will strengthen estrogen levels and fertile cervical mucous and therefore increase conception likelihood. When taken twelve hours after intercourse, it supports progesterone levels and behaves in the body much like the morning-after pill. Many women of childbearing age are successfully using Wild Carrot Seed as their primary method of contraception. A dear friend and herbalist shares that she used a combination of Wild Carrot and Mugwort (*Artemesia vulgaris*) during her perimenopause and enjoyed frequent intercourse through her fertile times and did not conceive.

My mother, who has a hot constitution and sleeps with the windows open even in the depths of winter, thoroughly enjoys the herb Damiana (*Turnera diffusa*) now that she has completed her journey through menopause. During the days of her hot flashes, she reported that Damiana would bring on the heat. Now, this can be person-specific—a woman who runs cold (or a man, for that matter)—can find this warming stimulant appealing regardless of phase of life. Damiana, with its warming, peppery flavor is a native to southwestern Texas and Mexico and is delightful in tea or tincture form—and commonly touted as an aphrodisiac aperitif. It is a member of the mint family and has a strong affinity for the pelvis. In fact, it specifically increases circulation to the nerves in the pelvic region.

Milky Oats, *Avena sativa*, is another fabulous lubricant along the nerves. The milky latex strengthens the myelin sheath that surrounds the nerves and improves electrical conductivity along those pathways. This milky substance is also lubricating to the mucous membranes of the reproductive and urinary tracts. The tincture of Milky Oats, taken in drop doses—between ten and thirty drops at a time, several times per day—coats and cools inflamed and brittle tissues and begins to strengthen them, while also improving the sensorial response to pleasant touch in the area. Among the first words of wisdom I learned about Milky Oats were, "It's fabulous for moistening mucous membranes, especially down there." This was coming from a gorgeous buxom woman in her forties in a handsome red dress, speaking in a sensual, seductive, confident tone of frank playfulness, "It gets you wet in almost an instant."

It's with a twinkle in my eye that I leave you with this fun bit of herbal exploration. May each step through fields, forest, desert, or along sidewalk connect you with the green plant blessings around you.

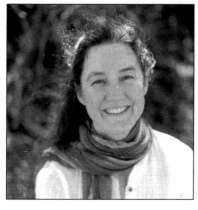

Mischa Schuler is a community herbalist and fertility awareness and shamanic practitioner in Portland, Maine, where she specializes in women's and children's health. Her herbal studies have been through apprenticeship with Deb Soule of Avena Botanicals, and clinically at the Tai Sophia Institute in Laurel, Maryland, where she earned a Master of Science degree in Herbal Medicine. Mischa offers apprenticeship programs and classes locally. Her greatest teachers are the plants and she feels tremendous gratitude that she is able to share their gifts through teaching, gardening, and in consultation.

Learn more: www.WildCarrotHerbs.com

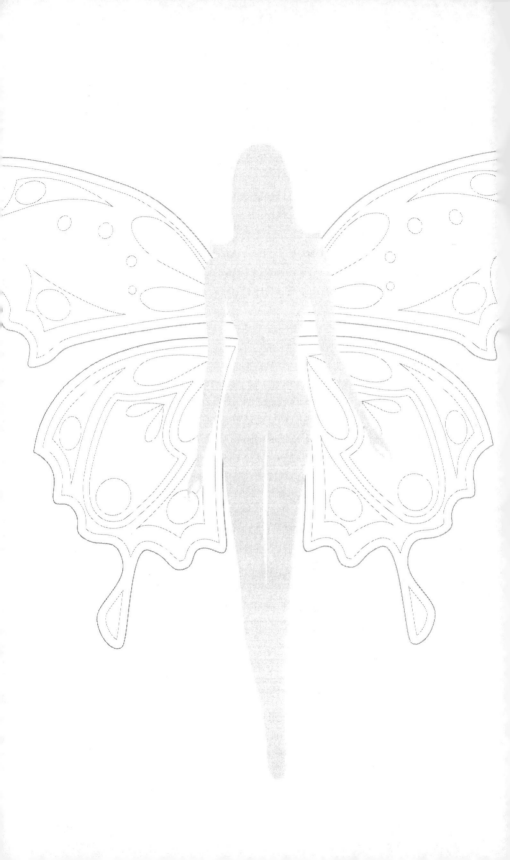

20

Menopause:
The Journey Back Home to Pure Love

MARY SHACKELFORD

Menopause is a time for awakening. It's a deep dive into a woman's heart, spirit, and true nature—that is, a time for pure love.

Menopause is a beautifully sacred time when we can take all the experiences of life—the journey so far—and go deeply within to release what is no longer needed. It is when we open ourselves to a new phase that has the potential to be a richer and deeper experience with more wisdom and inner truth… a deeper *knowing*.

It's a unique opportunity to open up to our heart in a deep way—to find what is true for us and to allow our own spirit and soul to truly flourish, allowing our wings to open and spread more fully.

This is not to say that we have not been our true self all along—we have. Yet this is a time to come full circle, to be whole, taking all that we have experienced, all our wisdom and knowing, and gathering it up, pulling it back together into our full self. It is a time to honor it all: the pain, the joy, the tears, and the laughter. We can see ourselves more clearly and hear our inner voice more loudly. That voice is no longer overshadowed by the innocence of youth, the fierceness of motherhood, or the boldness of building a career. It is stronger, yet *softer*.

Often in our society the experience of menopause is not portrayed as the incredible opportunity it is. Instead, it seems as if we cross over the forty threshold and things seem to take an abrupt turn to the south—literally and figuratively. Our body starts changing. Perhaps we bleed more or bleed less, our desire for sex changes, our body becomes softer, perhaps a little more plump and round.

Our relationships shift. Suddenly the house is quieter, or nearly silent. Our children leave the nest and embark on their own journey, leaving us behind a bit. The way we mother has to change. Sometimes we hold on really tight, in an attempt to be as much a part of their life as we were when they were toddlers. This rarely works out well for anyone involved!

We may feel a lack of intimacy and connection in our most beloved relationships. We may wonder where the spark went or if it is even still love.

Often we find ourselves feeling less than satisfied in our career, perhaps feeling bored or, just the opposite, tired of feeling constantly frazzled and time pressured.

We may even begin to notice an undercurrent of restlessness, a feeling of being unsettled, perhaps anxious or even jittery.

It's like the tectonic plates in our life have moved under us.

This experience can feel painful or unwanted. We don't really know what to do, which direction to go, where to start to feel solid ground underneath us again. It seems like everything is working against us—our body, our children, our partner, and even the career or profession we chose no longer feels right.

And so we begin to question who we really are, perhaps even thinking we are going a little crazy.

The years leading into "the change" were the most transformational of my life. In fact, I have come to know that the big change in my life had much less to do with my ovaries and their desire for a deep slumber than with *finding my heart* and what I truly love.

My journey into menopause began with quite a jolt. And in one single day, everything seemed to change. It happened in a blink of an eye and seemingly out of nowhere. It was supposed to be the first day of an incredible trip to Ireland for a vacation with my three sisters. Finally, some time away from work, time away from being a mom and wife—just me, my sisters, and a lot of fun.

On our transatlantic flight, I woke up with a pounding heart, nausea, sweaty palms, and an indescribable sense of impending doom and fear. I was overtaken by this physical response and a deep sense of dread.

As it turns out, I was having the first of many, many *panic attacks*. Prior to this event, my life seemed pretty normal. I was a working mom with a very busy, hectic job full of travel. I, like so many women, spent my day trying to keep all the balls in the air, making sure work projects were going the way they should (which never seemed to happen), keeping a home all while "being there" for my teenage kids and for my husband.

On the outside it all looked good: a great job with a significant salary, travel to beautiful cities, two amazing kids I adored, and a loving husband who even did laundry and helped with meals and the dishes.

Yet, on the inside, I was constantly struggling for a sense of control, to keep everything running, to keep everyone happy. Everyone except me, that is. It felt like if one thing got out of order, the whole day fell apart. I struggled to relax, to have fun, and to enjoy my life. I moved from one task to another endlessly.

At the time, I didn't realize the depths of the transformation I would undergo because of this one day. At that moment and for the next couple of years, in fact, I just felt suspended, held hostage by constant panic and fear. It was like my body and my mind were waging war on me.

After several months, I was continuing to have the attacks, often up to a dozen times a day. I was afraid that life as I knew it was over. I found myself dreading going places for fear of having an attack. I remember being in disbelief at how out of control, upside down, and weak I felt.

I couldn't believe this was how my life was going to end up. Me, feeling afraid to leave my house and even afraid to be *in* my house, living in fear all the time. I didn't even know what I was freaking afraid of! It was just fear with no rhyme or reason.

I knew deep inside the solution wasn't going to be found hiding out or in a pill bottle. My life had to change at a fundamental level.

Through what I now know was Divine intervention, I began to connect through books, workshops, friends, and Google searches with a new circle of teachers, doctors, and healers who were talking about the mind-body-spirit connection in ways that were new to me.

As I began to implement these natural and holistic practices—yoga, meditation, diet changes—the grip of the panic seemed to ease up. I felt a renewed sense of hope. Yet I still looked over my shoulder every day waiting for panic to show up again. And occasionally it would, each time leaving me in a bit of a tailspin for a few days.

As I continued with my fierce self-care, a deeper realization came to me. It was not enough to just take care of myself from a physical standpoint.

As beneficial as these practices were, they were often acting like a mere bandage—keeping the wound covered and protected, but the wound was still there. The wound I discovered was a soulful, spiritual one. I was living a life full of "shoulds," never allowing myself to really consider what my heart wanted, what *I* wanted at a deeper soul level. I was just doing what I thought I should in order to have what I thought I should have: a proper house, a fancy car, hundreds of pairs of shoes. I call it the "3P" disease—*People Pleasing Perfectionism.*

None of it was feeding *my soul* in the way it needed.

The real turning point came when I began to explore the concept of living with more awareness and seeing the world through the lens of love: Pure Love. I put that love into action through the passion coming from within my own heart and spirit.

I have come to believe that my journey to menopause was the path back to a deeper connection to myself. I was finally coming home.

Menopause forced me to pay attention to my body—my spirit's physical home—in a deeper way, to listen to the messages Spirit was sending me through my body.

What I have come to believe with all my being is that my body rose up in protest to living a life devoid of consciousness, connection to my heart and devoid of love in the forms of joy, fun, passion, and pleasure.

Panic sent a message I could not ignore to finally stop the madness, to let go of my people pleasing perfectionist ways and allow myself to listen to my heart and to my spirit for the first time *ever.*

Along the way I came to realize I had to be my own keeper, my own best friend. I had to start putting myself first. I had to take care of myself physically and spiritually. I had spent too many decades giving myself away—giving away my heart, my time, my love, my money, my compassion, my empathy, my sleep, my best ideas, and my creativity. I gave it away to my friends, boyfriends, husband, children, family, and job. Hell, my toilet got better care from me than what I gave myself.

I began exploring what it is I truly wanted. *Me.* Not what my husband wanted, my kids, my parents, or my fifth-grade teacher. Just me. I tuned in to what lit up my heart and what made me smile from the inside out and feel excited about my life, and the panic, anxiety, and stress dissipated. Once I really allowed myself to be first on the list, to speak my truth—to choose love and passion and pleasure every single day—panic was no longer needed. It had completed its mission of awakening me.

It has been a sweet journey of awakening—getting to know myself in a deeper way and allowing myself to experience life on my terms from a place of love. I am no longer compelled to play by the "rules" that squashed my spirit.

I discovered that when I show up fully as myself and give myself the space to discover who that even is my whole world is filled with the magic of life. I notice the colors that draw my eye and the textures that feel lovely against my skin. I notice the tastes that excite my mouth and leave it wanting more... the jokes and stories that make me laugh until I cry... the friends who warm my heart... my husband's touches that set me on fire... the sound of music that fills my ears, brings joy to my heart and entices my hips to sway to the beat. I am exploring it, feeling all of it—fully.

When I live this way, I am truly overflowing and I have more to give others.

We have been raised to believe that menopause is the beginning of the end, or perhaps even The End as we know it. And there is some loss, for sure, if you choose to see it that way. I say, give yourself permission to fully feel any of the losses you perceive. And then turn them around; find the gift.

We can decide to see menopause as an opportunity to fully come into ourselves as a woman experiencing this human life. This is the best time in our life to open our arms and our hearts to what is possible for us. We are in the prime time to create the life we dream of. We have experiences and wisdom to lean on. We are strong. We know the deepest depths of love. And we know how to create because we have been doing it our whole lives: not only creating new life, but creating projects and products and companies.

We can create an amazing second act by just shifting our perception from creating life outside ourselves to one of creating our life from the inside out.

I have come to know that following our heart and our passion is the key to navigating menopause. Doing this *is* "the Change." If we can begin to do more of that on a daily basis without guilt or self-judgment, the other experiences that come along with this time in our life seem much less bothersome or important. Having a hot flash while you are doing something you love is a completely different experience than when you are feeling miserable in your life.

Menopause is the beginning of stepping more fully into your body in a way you never could when you were twenty; of owning its feminine beauty and its power for pleasure; of standing tall and proud and open to the goddess energy that you are.

Along with the panic and anxiety, I have experienced many of the other usual suspects: hot flashes, heavy periods, bouts of anemia, night sweats, irritability, and weight gain. I have come to see the symptoms my body is experiencing as my barometer for living life in love, passion, and pleasure.

When I am hot flashing it's a message to check in and see what is "heating" me up and tune into what is underneath those flashes. Is it frustration? Fear? Anger? Boredom? Self-judgment? I know that often I use food—sugar and carbs—as a salve, and my body responds with more hot flashes to get my attention. I also find that when I am not feeling juicy and excited or experiencing much pleasure in my life, my body reflects that, too, and I am drier with less sexual desire and passion.

Menopause continues to be my teacher. My body reflects what's in my heart and my soul. It's my barometer of the love I am allowing in. When I wallow in worry and despair, my body withdraws, shrivels, and becomes less open for pleasure. But when I live in my heart and allow my passion to flow and seek pleasure daily, my body reflects a suppleness and openness to receiving physical love and pleasure.

The beauty of my menopause journey is realizing that it's my obligation to the world to put myself first, to show up as my true self. Otherwise I show up as a dulled, smaller version of myself. And we all lose.

My wish for you is Pure Love, to give yourself time and space to listen to your heart, to follow your passions and never settle for anything less than what feels good to you. Ever.

Once you fill yourself from your internal well of love, it cannot help but spill out into the world around you.

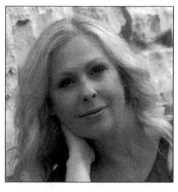

*Leadership requires vision, passion and bravery, qualities that **Mary Shackleford** found over a lifetime of happiness, meeting the obstacles blocking her path with her own evolutionary awareness. Even when her life was derailed by the specter of panic attacks and overwhelming fear, Mary sought answers and pushed forward, filled with the knowing that there was more to learn-the quiet intuition that love was the answer...*

Mary is taking a stand for pure love... and her business Pure Love Lifestyle reflects honesty, connection and flow—a lifestyle of passion and freedom from the choices and beliefs that no longer serve you. Pure Love is grabbing the tambourine of life and making music without judgement or rules. Love and laughter—intimacy and fearlessness. Giving with an open heart and receiving with joy... Pure love is presence and fire and radical responsibility.

With a career in nursing and multiple degrees and certifications in nutrition and coaching, Mary uses her skills and passions to create a pathway to positivity—a lifetime of searching uncovering the layers of darkness and finding the light burning bright within. Mary is ready to lead women back to their hearts, and the transformation of pure love.

*Learn more: **www.PureLoveLifestyle.com***

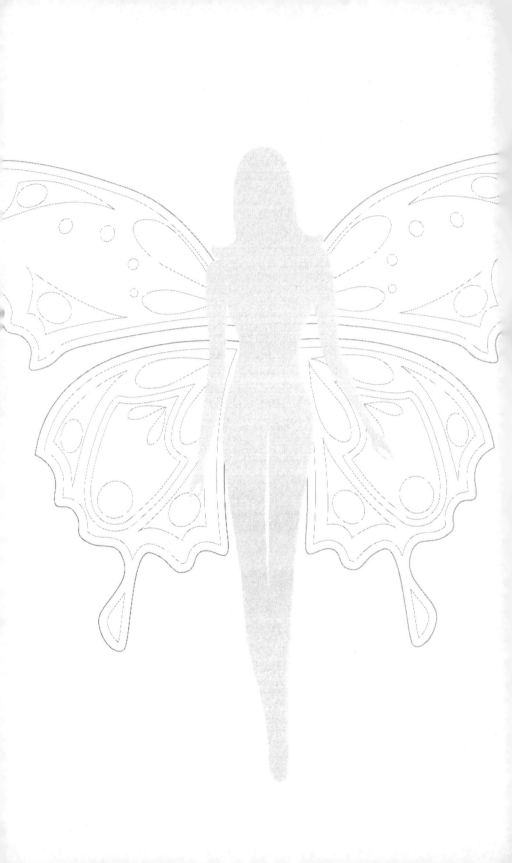

21

Align and Shine

CYDNEY SMITH

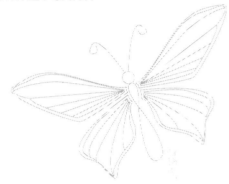

The teacher training room is full, and the asana practice has begun. I place my mat near the door and sit in meditation while others practice. My yoga today is to "be here." I feel too weak and vulnerable to do the vigorous sequence. As the class moves through the sequence, the room heats up, and I can feel the intense focus and the struggle to find ease. The teacher speaks to the class as they hold a pose, "There is nowhere to be but here. Accept where you are. Surrender to this moment. What is, is."

I push myself into a downward-facing dog pose, a resting pose I've done thousands of times. Another teacher, Bryan, comes to assist me, placing his hands firmly on mine holding my wrists. I stretch back into the pose and breathe, release. There is nowhere to be but here… accept… surrender… I find strength and surrender in the pose. The class shifts to the next pose, Bryan releases the assist, and I wobble. I try to hold the pose for a moment longer, and I have the thought I can't do it without support.

I realize this is true in my life right now. I don't have the strength to go on without support. The realization brings me to my knees, and tears begin to flow. I jump up and head for the door. I make it to the bathroom and cry. I want to leave; this isn't working, I'm not ready. And then I realize there's nowhere to be but here. If I leave, the feelings come with me.

I'd signed up for the yoga teacher training at my local yoga studio, something I'd wanted to complete for many years. My word for the year had been "alignment." I welcomed things that brought me a sense of being aligned with my truth, my authenticity, my vision and goals. The word became a question that I asked myself every day, "Do I feel in alignment with this?" Signing up for the training, the timing felt right.

After waiting a month to begin, it turned out timing wasn't quite right—at least not in the way I had originally thought. I had imagined myself serenely deepening my yoga practice, juicing, sweating, and balancing in crow and headstand… But coming into alignment turned out to mean something totally different for me. It seems that I had much deeper work to do and much bigger things to let go of then a little tension and a coffee habit.

The first weekend of the training I was only able to attend for the introductions and overview. I needed and wanted to get back to my house, to stay close to my husband Chris as he adjusted to being home and healing. A few weeks earlier, he had suffered a twenty-foot fall, broken bones, skull fracture, and a traumatic brain injury. He had just returned home after a week in ICU and an additional week on the special care floor for brain injuries. He was doing well, all things considered, and could function on his own. But he was not supposed to be left alone, as his day-to-day recovery was still unpredictable. My brother was staying with him that morning, but I was undone and not really in the frame of mind to attend a training.

To say I was out of alignment would be an understatement. Stress, fear, sleepless nights, a messy house, and worries about my husband, the future, the money, our kids, and the day-to-day recovery weighed on me. I had no filters; I was teary and unsure. The accident had stopped me in my tracks. When something traumatic happens, everything else falls away—or seems to. Really, "everything else" is just lurking on the sidelines, becoming a mess, like a garden left untended with the weeds still growing. It's still there when you are ready to for it. At some point it comes back into focus, and the time and energy to clean it up is unexpected

Over the course of that first month after the trauma, Chris shifted from critical care to stabilizing in a private room and then home with visiting nurses. The focus from the critical moment to moment began to shift and I felt my world begin to crash. I had been buoyed by the adrenaline of crisis, by living in the reality of doctors and tests, and sleeping the final days in his private room at the hospital. But once we got home, I began to panic and feel overwhelmed by all the day-to-day upheaval. In addition to Chris's care, I began to cave under the circumstances of a life untended.

I remember the moment of feeling like I was a sinking ship—I had only $50 cash available to me, though I knew a little money would arrive Friday from my consulting work. Friends had set up a meal train, and lovingly prepared meals were being dropped off three nights a week. Another friend had brought a bag of groceries with food for our daughters' lunches and snacks. In the meantime, power and gas had gone off—and been turned back on—as the mail sat neglected. The water heater valve broke and flooded the base-ment. The sink was leaking. I was at the grocery store, with a $50 bill in my back pocket, not wanting to risk messing up the delicate balance of my low bank account. I was focusing on what I needed to get through the week, how to do it on $50, and trying not to think about next week or the future.

At the register, I reached into my pocket—and it was empty. Fear drained me in that moment, and I meekly said I needed to check my car. It wasn't there. I got in the car about to drive away, ready to give up and resigned to go down with the ship. In that moment I felt ashamed, depressed, saddened and, ultimately, a victim of tragedy, circumstance, and my own failures and inadequacies.

I sat for a moment more, then mustered up courage, probably for my children. I walked back in to the store, wanting proof that things were going to be okay. I wanted proof to trust, have faith, and believe it would be okay. I stopped at the customer service desk, and was given an envelope with my $50 dollar bill, handed in by "a nice young man." I bought my groceries for $38 and drove away.

Shaking and crying, I pulled into the Starbucks drive-thru. Should I? I could go home and make a coffee… but I wasn't ready to go home yet. At the pick-up window, I was told that my coffee had already been paid for. As I let that incredible coincide sink in, my phone rang. I had gotten into a habit of not answering unless the call was from a doctor. But I answered, and it was my friend Betsy from California. Feeling slightly elated, half laughing, half crying, I told her about the grocery store and the coffee.

With concern she asked, "Do you need money? Are you letting people help you? I know you must have lots of people who want to help." I told her about the meals, and the many, many offers for support and help.

She persisted.

"But I just don't know what I need," I replied, meekly.

"You need to say 'Yes' to every offer that comes your way, whether you think you need the help or not," Betsy told me. "Let people help you. I know you are capable and strong, but this is hard enough. Let other people take care of themselves. If they are offering, they want to help."

"I feel like such a taker," I said, beginning to cry. "I don't want to take things from people."

"Oh my God, you are not taking anything! People are giving. They are offering. Change the word. You are a receiver. People are giving because they want to help and support you."

It was my wake-up call. I don't recall what or how I said yes over those next few weeks and months, but miracles happened. Chris continued to recover. Fundraisers were set up. Checks arrived in the mail via the fundraiser, and balances were paid: my daughters' extracurricular activities, school tuition, oil for the winter, and rent were paid. Leaves were raked, children were driven to activities, dinner continued to be dropped off, even by restaurants from a friend afar. I received a massage, facials, and lots of hugs, texts, and calls. A steady stream of love poured in.

And a funny thing happened. I broke open. It was so overwhelming, so humbling, and so necessary it brought me to my knees. The gratitude that filled me, and still does, stripped away pretenses of what should be, of how I thought I should be, and I saw what was really important to me. I recognized that even at my weakest and most vulnerable, I was worthy of love and support. My future—my family's future—would be okay, and I could choose to believe that.

I returned to my mat, where I sat and cried.

"Accept where you are," the instructor told the class. "Surrender. There is no place to be but here. What is, is."

I cried, shook, breathed. I sat with my fear, anger, grief, vulnerability, and gratitude. All of it. And began to release. Letting go of all expectations of what I should be, what my life should be, and what I thought I should be doing. Letting go of disappointment and self-judgment and recognizing that my fear lived there. I breathed in love, and released fear on the out breath. No matter where I go, my feelings go with me, so I might as well feel them. I chose to accept support—to heal, and to move forward with an open heart of gratitude—even while crying and feeling vulnerable.

When my cousin Therese called me the week before Christmas, I told her about the yoga training.

"That's good you're doing it this year," she said. "You need it for you. You've got to take care of you so you can take care of that man of yours and those beautiful babies. I want to give you something, and I don't want you to say no. Just tell me who to call. I want to get you a facial or massage. You are important, too."

I messaged her the information, and I thanked her.

"How will I ever pay everyone back?" I asked.

"You pay it forward by being you. You have a long life to pay it forward. Sometimes just being who you are is enough. People want to help you and your family."

I made the choice to begin to move forward by enjoying the holidays. I spent a week with Chris, our girls, and our family. I had fun, rested, and felt ready to head home and get some ground under my feet. I had work to do and I felt that familiar desire to take charge and get it done coming back to me. I would move forward and let myself be at my best. Being vulnerable and needing help didn't have to mean being a victim, giving up, or being less than. My worth was not attached to my circumstances. The best way I could pay it forward, be grateful, and say thanks was by getting back on my feet to take care of myself.

To come into alignment with myself I needed to let go of the stuck energy that had developed in my early forties. For a few years before Chris's accident, I had felt out of sorts, like I couldn't get my mojo going. I still had young kids. There was a recession, we downsized, lost work and a business, and we went on living our lives and raising kids. Things didn't always look great, but they weren't all that bad, either. And yet I had begun living from disappointment instead of living from possibility. Perhaps that's the midlife crisis. The melancholy that comes from living a full life, taking care of others and forgetting to connect with our own passions and purpose. We come out of alignment, spending too much time on certain aspects of our lives, neglecting others.

I'm a wellness coach and entrepreneur who has a solid understanding of anatomy, biology, and physiology. I had a base knowledge of hormones, aging, wrinkles, hot flashes, sleepless nights, and moodiness. But, somehow, I didn't give too much thought to menopause, figuring I'd cross that bridge when I got there. But suddenly here I was, waking up to precursors of "the change," but not knowing what it meant. I recognized myself getting older. My friends began to talk about aging and lost youth. I saw that movie stars who were my age now played the parents and even they—professionals who were paid to look good—were aging. Looking back, there were physical signs, too. But they were subtle, almost too subtle to distinguish from moments caused by that lack of self-care. Was I pushing myself too much and not sleeping enough? Was I drinking too much coffee, eating gluten and dairy? Too much red wine? Is that why I felt tired, bloated, cranky, and had trouble sleeping? Maybe it was my career, marriage, finances, dreams not yet realized? Who could tell?

Was it coincidence or synchronicity that I had such a stark opportunity to reexamine my life at age forty-five? That my word for that year was "alignment"? This year is the point at which one chapter ended… and another began.

For me, change has always come swiftly, like a flood ripping through the landscape. It leaves everything in its wake bare, ravaged and upturned. The secret of the flood is that it creates fertile ground for new growth. Having carried minerals and nutrients from afar, the flood deposits them on bare soil. I had experienced the chaos of crisis and the hyper-focus that comes with it. Now, having it stripped away, I began to see the life I love and witness the foundation of who I am. I felt the deep feeling of gratitude that this moment, this life, is full of possibility.

This is alignment—myself stripped of all the shoulds, the stories of what I think is or isn't. How much of our daily suffering, aches, and pains come from the stories we tell ourselves about our lives?

In her book *The Wisdom of Menopause*, Dr. Christiane Northrup, says that pre-menopause is a time to create a life you want and that we are actually coming home to ourselves. She addresses the myths of midlife—that it is a downward spiral for women—instead calling it an actual renaissance of our lives. I had been reaching, trying to grab hold of what I had thought was slipping away from me physically. But, even more so, I was attached to a sense of failure for not being what I thought I should be or wanted to be. All along, I had been reaching outside myself and believing that I couldn't or wouldn't be enough. Thoughts of failure were fueling my aging, fueling my perception of time slipping away

Now, I am embracing this new chapter of my life. Instead of reaching for the past, or grasping to the future out of fear, I am deepening into myself. Much like my yoga poses, as I deepen, I strengthen and align. The lesson for me is to be grateful for the moments of life. To stop reaching and to deepen, to breathe and to learn to hold the pose, the moment, a little longer. To breathe into my life and do more of what I love and less looking for what I love. As I practice, I come closer to my own possibility and alleviate the suffering of thinking I am anything other than this experience, this moment. At times, a guiding hand to assist and a firm grip of support are welcomed and needed. Each day I begin again, learning to be present to myself at this moment, in this life.

My dear cousin Therese passed away unexpectedly a few days after Christmas. She was only fifty-four. She was a lively, much-loved fiery red-head who brought laughter wherever she went. As I move forward and pay it forward, I hear the priest talking about her namesake, St. Therese, who had announced her vocation as love. St. Therese had carried out small, daily acts of love in devotion to a power greater than herself. I'll remember Therese this way as well.

I will continue to grow and change and pursue my dreams, ambitions, and passions. In honoring my cousin Therese, I will seek to love what is more, focusing on living instead of what is dying. But deepening into my life, I become the best expression of me there is. I recognize that being myself allows me to pay it forward and contribute to the very fabric that supported me, to be part of something larger, to be part of my community and family. To shine.

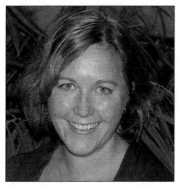

Cydney Smith is a bit of a wellness cowgirl offering programs that inspire an independent and bold approach to your own health and happiness. Look for the next step of your wellness journey over at SpiritedNutrition.com. She lives with her husband and two daughters in southwestern New Hampshire.

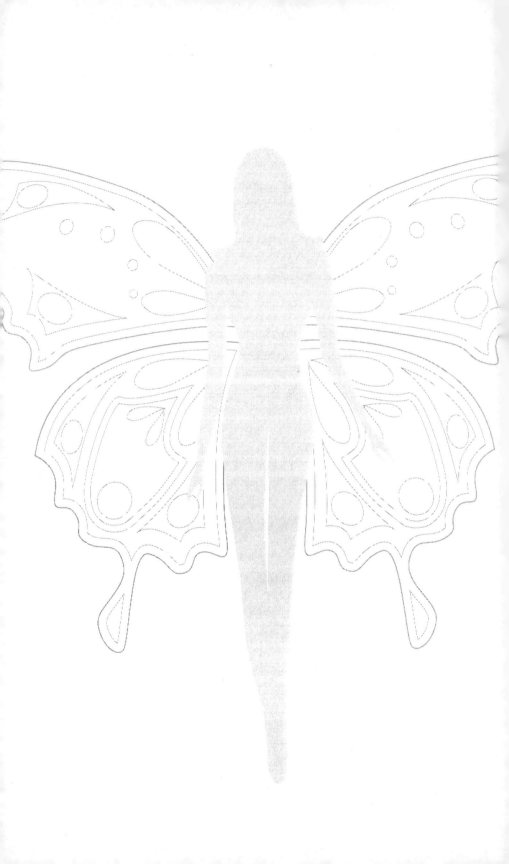

22

Deeply Rooted Trees

SAGE SOLIS

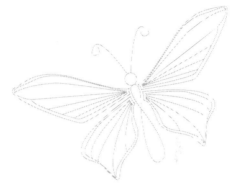

Older trees are deeply rooted into the earth. They are tall and able to withstand the seasons and most weather conditions. As a tree grows tall, so does its roots, intertwined far below the earth. A lifetime of seasons have strengthened her for the rest of her journey. A menopausal woman is like this deeply rooted tree. She, too, has withstood many seasons. Her wisdom is at its peak. She is stronger now and more powerful and can use this new tool to improve her life. Margaret Mead once said, "There is no more creative force in the world than a menopausal woman with zest." If we decide to use our menopausal powers, this zest that she speaks of is the result of this decision.

This chapter is about finding your zest so you can transcend and grow as a woman faster than you ever have before. I will walk you down the path of my story and then introduce you to the first step of transcending through menopause. This step is very important because it forces you to make a choice. The last part of the chapter is about the gifts of menopause and how to use them as your super fuel to grow and transcend as a woman.

Menopause is the death of our fertility, but it is also the birth of a new chapter of our life as women. When we learn that we are in menopause, the first thing we do is go into denial. Denial is normal—it's the first stage of grief, and we are most certainly grieving. Second, we are totally thrown off of our cycle that we have relied on for decades. Over the years as we ovulate and bleed, we come to rely on this cycle. But when menopause hits, it's like we're suddenly and harshly thrown out of the four seasons and into perpetual winter without a choice. We may spend the first year of menopause not only in denial but in a new season that never ends. Everything in our body changes, just like it did in puberty, and it takes a while to come to terms with this new cycle of living. Once the grieving is over, the magic can start to happen and the blooming of new and even more beautiful parts of ourselves can shine through.

In May 2012, I had one of my last periods of my life. I didn't know it was one of my last periods, or maybe I would have enjoyed it a little bit more. There is something very comforting about spending a week, cramping to various degrees, feeling hormonal. For me, the cycle is like the four seasons where the period is symbolic of winter. It represents death, and regeneration to follow the next month—like Shiva the destroyer. We dive deep into our psyche, figure out all that is wrong in our world, and deal with it, destroy it, and then regenerate the next month. We take it for granted most of the time. Looking back, I counted on my monthly cycle to guide me through my life. My dear friend Ami, who worked with me for years, used to tell me that she liked it when I had PMS because I got everything done (personally and professionally) during that week. She was right.

At first, I enjoyed not having periods. After a while though, I started to question it. I was only forty-five. It seemed too soon. I'd had a miscarriage the year before. In my mind, I was still fertile. I scheduled an appointment with my gynecologist, who informed me that I was in menopause. I was not perimenopausal; I was completely menopausal. She explained to me that menopause can come as early as forty-five—it is rare, but it happens. I left the office bewildered. I told everyone. I remember not really getting any reaction from anyone. They looked at me blankly, with a look that said, "I have no idea what you are talking about." So, I continued on with my period-less life and totally forgot that I was in menopause. Denial can be quite powerful.

As the months went on, I started getting panic attacks again. I was immersed in an advanced training with my yoga teacher and was taking it *much* too seriously. I was feeling crankier than normal. I started getting hot flashes. All this was going on and it never occurred to me that this had anything to do with menopause. In fact, I was in total denial. I honestly thought I could get pregnant again, even though my doctor told me my chances of getting pregnant were less than 0.5 percent.

My body started giving up on me. I went to the ER because my hands and feet were numb and I couldn't breathe—it turns out I was having a massive panic attack. Later, I was diagnosed with diverticulitis. I severely sprained my ankle. I presented with an ulcer. And, finally, I injured my back—all this in the span of a year.

During the peak of my menopause experience, my husband was offered a job on the other side of the country. We knew right away that this was his dream job and we were going to move. But the stress of it all sent me over an edge that I had never been over before. Suddenly, everything was a big deal to me. It seemed that my emotions were heightened 1000 percent. Saying goodbye to each friend in California, one after the other for weeks on end, sent me into tears every day. Moving became my full-time job. I was hyper-obsessed with everything: finding the best school, finding the best house, staying on budget, having a great relationship with my husband, *and* being the best mom throughout the entire process.

By the time we got to New Jersey, I felt like I had been fighting in the trenches. I was worn out mentally—like I used to feel when I was an ICU nurse. Little did I know that the journey was not over. We stayed in temporary housing for over a month waiting to close on our new home. We ate out every day. I had recently gained 10 pounds, and now, without a kitchen, I put on another 10 pounds. I knew my health was declining. My clothes didn't fit. I could barely walk up the stairs. My ankle hurt 24/7. So I found a new primary care doctor that was a D.O. He spent over an hour with me going over my symptoms, my weight, and my stress level.

He looked me straight in the eyes and said, "All of these things you have gone through over the past year are due to menopause. You are hormonally out of sorts and the stress is exacerbating your ulcer and diverticulitis." He told me that women who go into menopause early tend to experience it more intensely. He recommended that I see a gynecologist right away. I went home completely overwhelmed. I knew that I would never be able to take hormonal therapy because of my family history of breast cancer.

The good news was that I was finally understanding and accepting that I was in menopause. Looking back now, I can see why my panic attacks came back, why the ulcer would not heal, and why the diverticulitis kept acting up. I was overly stressed. My life had changed. I had moved across the country, which is one of the most stressful events of anyone's life. But something else had changed. My hormonal shift was allowing me to really *feel* everything. My health was screaming at me and so was my soul and the message that it was telling me was, "Alert, Alert, Alert!" The message was *so* loud that I medicated myself and did all the wrong things for my ulcer, my ankle, my diverticulitis. I was a mess and couldn't see a light at the end of the tunnel. As it turns out, I was in the middle of a dark night of the soul—a depression. I was numbing out, self-medicating, and finding any way possible to *not* look at my issues.

This whole thing was a conundrum for me. My life was good! I had everything I needed, including a great family and amazing people surrounding me. But when menopause hit, it was like PMS x 1000. Everything that was wrong, sad, or scary was completely magnified. At the time, I thought that this was a bad thing because my pain was so amplified, but I have since learned the greatest truth about menopause. This was a blessing—because when I was waking up at 3 a.m. every day, my alert button was going off and telling me *exactly* what was bothering me. I had two options: take sleeping pills or deal with what was keeping me up.

I chose to deal with it.

TRANSCENDING

When we go into menopause we have to make a choice. You can deal with the issues bothering you, or you can bury your head in the sand.

Let me tell you about what happened with my parents over the summer.

My parents are divorced, but both of them wanted to come and see our new home. I set up a visit in which they would both be here at overlapping times. It turned out really well. We all had a good time, and it was healing in a way for me that I had not expected. After going to bed that first night they were here, I woke up—just like clockwork—at 3 a.m. What was bothering me on this particular night was that I was afraid that this would be the end of having them under one roof. Would this be the last time? What will I do if they died? How would I go on? I love them so much—and then the "aha" moment came. *I love them. I really, really, really love them so much that I could just lay in between them forever in eternal bliss.* What a beautiful feeling to discover within myself.

The 3 a.m. wakeup call was my gift. Once I identified what it was, I looked at it intensely, turned it inside out, and went back to sleep. I admitted my deepest fear—that that my parents would die—and then made the conscious choice to accept that and love them as hard as I could for the remainder of my life. I went back to sleep and slept like a baby.

We really had a wonderful visit. My mom and I unpacked boxes while my dad watched TV. We got in the hot tub, we swam, we went on long drives, we did puzzles, we ate out almost every night, and when we cooked, we laughed. I will cherish that visit for the rest of my life. I promised myself that I would spend the remainder of my parents' time on earth loving and doting on them. And now, I never wake up worrying about them dying anymore. I dealt with it. I made the decision to walk toward love and walk away from fear.

So, why is every issue you come across in menopause such a big deal? My theory is in mid-life our soul is screaming loudly to get our attention and heal what needs to be healed.

Transcending is a process in which we stop identifying with the lower Self (the physical body/ego) and start identifying with the higher Self (that is connected to your Eternal Soul, God, the Universe and all other beings). When we go into menopause, we have the choice to use the gifts that menopause brings and transcend, or continue to identify with only the lower Self. If we choose to identify with the lower Self, our perception of life is very self-centric and our perception of aging is of limitation—that it's the end of the road for us.

If we look at it as a gift and begin to start identifying with the higher Self, we are acknowledging that God is in all of us. We are understanding that we are all one.

Our decisions come from a place of unconditional love, compassion, awe-inspiring beauty and wisdom.

MENOPAUSE AS A PATH FOR TRANSCENDENCE

So how do we transcend through menopause? We listen to our soul. When we find ourselves in a situation that stresses us out, we listen to what our soul is telling us. Do we fear for a family member and the choices they are making? Do we fear that our lover is cheating on us? Do we feel upset because someone in our life is unkind? Whatever is waking you up in the night or is eating at you, address it. It all comes down to love. Love is all encompassing. This means that even fear is an aspect of love. So if you feel fear, turn the fear around into love. Instead of yelling at the person or crying over the pain or the fear, address it with love. Express your love to your friends and family.

In *A Course in Miracles,* the Introduction states, "The opposite of love is fear, but what is all-encompassing (love) can have no opposite." So what's waking you up at 3 a.m.? LOVE. It is your soul crying, "You are in menopause my dear, your life is halfway over. Deal with it!" Turn it inside out and into love. This is our time to be wise and rise above our problems. You are a tall and deeply rooted tree now that continues to be vibrant and alive. You are deeply rooted, because you have many years of life experience behind you. Your tree is tall and strong. It cannot be blown over. We are stronger than we have ever been, and we can handle it. Now is the time.

23

Luxury for Your Soul

JULIETTE TAYLOR-DE VRIES

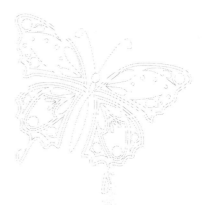

There are only two mistakes one can make along the road to truth; not going all the way, and not starting.

—The Buddha

Imagine jumping out of bed and into your life with excitement and enthusiasm.

Imagine having the unparalleled opportunity to completely transform your life

Imagine being in complete alignment within yourself.

I'd love to sit here and tell you that transforming your life into one you actually love is about inspiration, visualizing what it looks like when you're there, and acting as if you're already there. Although those are important components, they are not the foundational pieces to transformation. Strategy and action are the pillars to transformation, and both require taking a leap of faith, with an openness to taking on risks and becoming an investor in your happiness and future success.

When I turned forty, I truly understood what great dames of the past have repeated as a mantra and a call to action—that once you turn forty you stop caring about what others think of you. You start living your life on your own terms with no regrets. And I have to agree.

At forty I found my voice and then promptly lost it again at forty-one. In looking back I can only attribute it to fear. It's really scary to stand on the ledge and do what your gut, heart, and soul are begging you to do. It's really scary to trust that the universe will provide, that the unmanifest will be manifest, and that your thoughts and intentions will actually create a life you love. As freeing as it seems to stand in the space between the past and the future, it's much easier to swallow freedom, box it up, and place it somewhere in your deepest caverns. Yep, it's easier… but it sure creates havoc on your soul.

I know. I've been there done that and can say I've come out on the other side a little worn for the wear but unscathed. There is no bitterness to what I gave up in exchange for freedom. What I gave up was a big house on the shore, a yacht club membership, annual trips to Europe and the Caribbean, the Platinum soon to be the Black card, two six-figure incomes, and the storybook that I manifested. Even as I appeared to be living such a perfect life, something very deep was gnawing at me—that in order to manifest a spiritual and connected life, I had to give it all up. I had to jump before I could see the net and the path beyond. I had to trust the universe and myself like never before.

No, I'm not bitter. I'm elated and curious, I'm living in the moment, and I'm connected to the Divine. I have come out on the other side and embrace what it means to be a wise woman, a crone in the traditional witchy way. How did I do it? How do you do it?

We're all familiar with the Wheel of Life in coaching terminology, using the wheel to create a visual of where you are at the moment in relation to where you want to be. After lining up where each segment of my life was on the wheel, I could see that my wheel was a jagged trainwreck. None of the segments were the same size. My inner life was certainly not aligned with my outer life. And that needed to change.

The Wheel of Life I created is a bit different from others because it connects with the elements, our five senses, and to the chakras.

I welcome you to use Your Wheel of Life to gauge where you are right now—not in five minutes or in your mind—but where you are right now, this very moment, to where you want to be. Because where you are now isn't where you have to be.

The wheel is made up of the following slices.

PHYSICAL BODY (EARTH)—

Start Mindful Thinking: Hold yourself accountable, think about the actual words you are using. Words carry energetic vibrations and affect your cells, your body, perception, and the world around you. Deepak Chopra talks about this, about how when you say you have a heavy heart, if scientists looked inside they'd find it affected by molecules that cause stress and damage, such as excessive amounts of cortisol and adrenaline. Likewise, if you say you're bursting with joy, analysis would find your skin loaded with neuropeptides that may work like antidepressants.

EMOTIONS (WATER)—

Explore Your Story: Who are you? This is the first step to finding out who you are and what you are meant to do—your soul's purpose and destiny. Don't regret the past or fear the future.

MISSION AND PURPOSE (FIRE)—

Keep a Journal: Writing is the single-most important tool in accessing and crystallizing the thoughts and beliefs that ultimately lead to actions. If you don't write it down you haven't given birth to your dreams, your actions, and your best life ever. You haven't charted your course because you don't really know where you are going; you're jumping from one drama to another, one reaction to another. Accessing our thoughts and beliefs that drive our actions is the key component to unlocking the true and best you, creating sustainable and transformative change.

RELATIONSHIPS (AIR)—

Breathe: Actively breathe and do it consciously. Take a deep breath in, counting to eight. Breathe out, counting to four, and then breathe in again, counting to eight.

FINANCES (SOUND)—

Mantras and Affirmations: Say a mantra and hold that thought throughout the day.

SPIRITUALITY (SIGHT)—

Begin a meditation routine: Our intuition, or our sixth sense, taps directly into the Universe and Spirit guides us during those quiet moments. Start with a few minutes the same time every day and then add some minutes every week. Allow the Universe to speak to you.

GRATITUDE AND GIVEBACK (FEEL)—

Pray: Talk to Spirit/God/Divine. This is talking to the Universe.

Express Gratitude: Focus on what's good in your life and ask for more of it: We spend a lot of energy focusing on what's wrong with our lives or what we lack. Doing so only adds more of it as the Universe only understands how to give you more of what you ask for.

TIME (TOUCH)—

Take time during your day, preferably the same time every day for the same amount of time. Creating a space for rituals creates a space for the Universe to do her work and give you clues to the next steps through coincidences, hints, and synchronicity.

Rinse. Repeat for 12 months. It's okay to start with three months, because that's how long it takes to make or break a habit. Whether it's three months or a full year, your life will change, you'll reduce your stress levels, and you'll create a haven for intuition by learning to trust your instincts (and learning what that instinct feeling actually feels like in your body) and then using that intuitive sense in your day-to-day life. This process is paramount for any lasting success.

I started that process as a last-ditch effort when my internal life was spiraling out of control. Nobody else could see the internal chaos because on the outside my life looked as near as perfect as could be. It was time to get real with aligning the inner me with the outer me and then make a commitment to be willing to release all that didn't fit anymore. And so the following four phases ensued.

PHASE 1: DISCOVER YOUR INNER CORE

To create a life of extraordinary meaning, purpose, and fulfillment

PHASE 2: UNLOCK YOUR POTENTIAL

To discover what you want and how to get it

PHASE 3: REACH YOUR PINNACLE

To transform your emotions, health, relationships, and finances

PHASE 4: ACTIVATE YOUR PERSONAL BLUEPRINT

To determine the final integration

Implementing theses these four phases creates a holistic culture of quality—luxury for your soul. What I found is that my core values are just that—*core* values—and they are non-negotiable.

Here's my manifesto:

I preserve my quality of life by vibrating at the frequency of love.

I create a haven for intuition and following it—no matter what; I insist on leadership, friendships, and intimate relationships that are rooted in authenticity and clarity.

I live my life in a heart-centered way and am financially rewarded because compassion and capitalism can meld.

I make magical and electric atmospheres everywhere I go.

I give back.

And lastly, like Dolly Parton so eloquently quipped, I insist that you "get down from that cross, people need that wood for fire."

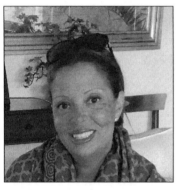

Juliette Taylor-De Vries guides women to find their path to cups-of-coffee-on-the-veranda-in-the-silence-of-the-morning kind of happiness, their path to unrelenting joy, and their path to contentment that's contagious. Creating LifesPath ™, the single most comprehensive path to health, happiness, and love, she has guided hundreds of clients to breakthrough their blocks by disproving the beliefs about themselves that are holding them back, to find the strength to live lives they want to wake up to each morning.

She helps clients maintain focus and attention on goals by creating successful routines that include powerful visualizations, calming meditations practices, daily spiritual/mindfulness rituals, and embracing a plant-based diet. Her approach isn't about eating well or meditating daily; it's about the whole package. Because she believes all are multidimensional, the perfect approach is multifaceted.

Juliette holds a BA from the University of California, Irvine; a Certificate in Plant-Based Nutrition from Cornell University; and a master's in Spiritual Metaphysics from the American Institute of Holistic Theology.

Her book The Four Tenets of Love *is available to order on her website www. juliettetaylor.com and at your local Barnes & Noble stores.*

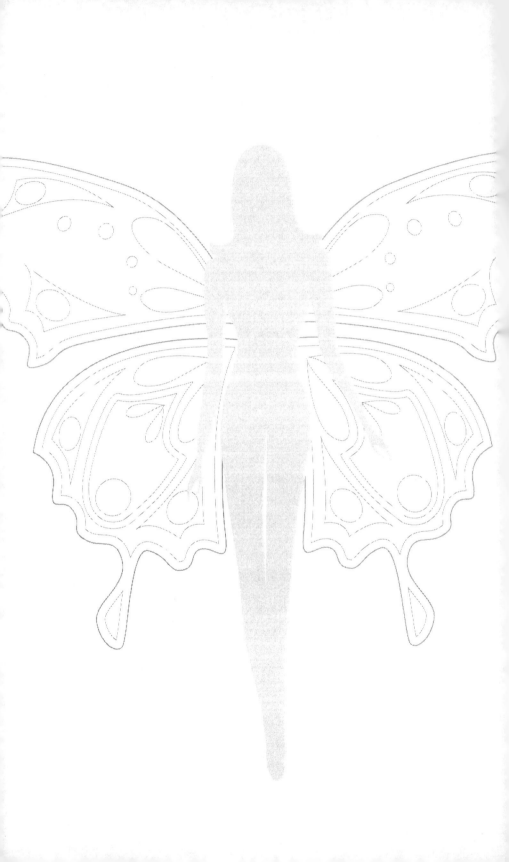

24

Dancing Through Menopause

LINDA VETTRUS-NICHOLS

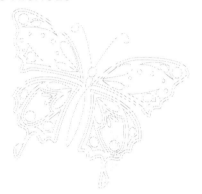

"The only way to make sense out of change is to plunge into it, move with it, and join the dance."

—Alan Watts

On my journey through menopause I came to understand the dance of the enlightened woman. During menopause, I learned that through the depths of the female psyche comes some of our greatest knowing. We can live fully present and aware of our psychic life or we can choose to be a victim of it, blaming others for our actions and reactions. After leaving a "starter marriage" of thirty-three years and finding the love of my life, I realized that the true love of my life was *me*. I am now a woman filled with *LaDestina*, a sense of my own destiny.

For decades, two major events had been dancing around in my head: the first was the tragic loss of my father, and the other was a physical accident that threatened my dance career.

My father was the hero in my life. We made dollhouse furniture together, and he was always available to watch the latest dance or gymnastics routine I had choreographed. One day just before starting my senior year of high school, I was babysitting for a neighbor, and the doorbell rang. When I opened the door and saw my uncle standing there, I knew something was not right. My uncle told me he would watch the kids and that my grandfather was at my house and my mother wanted to tell me something and my stomach began to churn. I was home in two seconds but it felt like I was moving through sludge. As I slowly opened the door I could hear my mother crying. My brother was crying too. I threw a look of "what is going on" at my grandfather. He proceeded to tell me he had found my father when he arrived at work. He had hung himself in the garage of my grandfather's janitorial service. Rather than going into shock or even crying, I became the "strong one."

My delayed grief caught up with me a month after burying my father. A friend of mine came over, flying up the steps screaming, "Linda, Linda, Linda, guess what?" I gasped for air, froze, and then I began to cry. All I could think was, "Oh, no! What else has happened? I can't take anything else!" I had just been spending hours sitting in my father's closet, smelling his clothes and thinking of our sacred times together. My friend was so sorry she had upset me. Later, she felt horrible when she found out that I had cried for two weeks after her visit until my mother sent me to see a pastor at our church whose wife had committed suicide.

That was an interesting yet very healing visit with that pastor. We just sat next to each other on the couch. We could feel the energy of respect for each other's journey, the loss, the wonderful memories we possessed, and the healing we were both receiving—similar to how reading this book will help others on their journey through a magical, yet bittersweet, time of transformation.

The next event happened a few months later. I was on track to become a professional dancer. I had joined the gymnastics team and had promised my dance teacher that I would stay off the equipment. But I caved into a request from my gymnastics coach and agreed to do a simple routine on the balance beam. I ended with a roundoff dismount. Unfortunately, I didn't know that the girl ahead of me had slid the mat, exposing a metal foot of the beam. I broke my heel and my ankle shifted, resting bone on bone.

I was told that I would never dance again, and, in fact, I would be lucky if walked. I certainly would never be able to tolerate an eight-hour rehearsal as a professional dancer. Well, I proved them wrong—I did walk, and even danced again.

All this pain, in such a short period of time, was triggered again when I hit menopause. I now understand that through the depths of the female psyche comes some of our greatest knowing. We can live fully present and aware of our psychic life, or we can choose to be a victim of it, blaming others for our actions and reactions. There is a gift in every challenge, and the beauty of menopause for me is how it became the portal for my own transformation.

Even though I got stuck many times along the way, I eventually discovered and embodied seven spiritual truths that can reduce the emotional pain that can come up during the menopausal years. Living fully present from your soul is about noticing what is coming up for you as your body and mind begin to shift. The following truths help me to dance in my own flow. They are the spiritual truths that I teach my clients to see what is really important to them and to be inspired by their own dance, getting them in touch with who they really are. I invite you to experience the gifts in all of them.

Reclaim the REAL you. Your soul knows who you are and why you are here. You are not here to heal but to remember. We all come from the same source. We have forgotten who we are and why it is important to encourage one another. Together we complete each other and that which is to be remembered. This, in turn, creates clarity. You are the unstoppable you. By listening to your soul you will know when you are DONE with a marriage, a job, a lifestyle, or even an addiction.

Stand in YOUR truth. There is great emotional freedom in living and standing in your truth. "I think" … "I can't" … "I don't know"— they're all lies. Stand in your truth and start living out your own civic engagement. Make a difference. We're not born to be alone. We are born to be seen and understood—and to love ourselves so we can love others in our community. At the end of the day, it's not what you are but *who* you are. Be genuine, be real, be authentic, and be in the moment. Feed your own soul first, and you will be successful in your own eyes as well as in the eyes of others.

Open YOUR receiving channels. When we are stressed we tend to push out, interrupt, and start thinking of what we will say next. Taking a breath helps us to open and receive what the other person is saying. Self-care is another way to open our receiving channels. When we don't feel well supported it's typically because we are not taking care of ourselves. You can share the load by delegating to others.

Pay attention to YOUR creative patterns. What do you do that gets your creative juices flowing? What is your tempo? What "costume" are you wearing today? Is it the one that serves you, allows you to feel and be yourself as you tune into your own vibrations? Create, understand, and pattern your inner peace by starting with yourself.

Know YOUR vision. Dreams that come true have plans, and plans are supported by goals. Setting a goal is about setting an intention. Taking consistent action and attaining small goals builds confidence. Lack of self-worth and self-confidence results in a "lack mentality." If you are coming from a place of lack, you are actually lowering the vibration of the planet. You will never know your vision until you reach out and help others. They will point out your gifts and what you did to really help them. What energy moves you forward? What excites you to do and be more than you are today?

Serve yourself FIRST. On an airplane we are taught to put on our own oxygen mask first so we can safely help others. When we put the needs of others first, we have less energy to help them. This way of life can also lead us into a "dis-ease" state. There is a price to pay living from such a place.

Know your REAL love. It's not about finding the love of your life; it's about finding you and loving you. Only then can the love of your life appear. This will empower you to love your life no matter what. If you have a man who loves you unconditionally, you are doing the same for yourself. If you have a man who never puts you down and feels you are "just right" or the "perfect fit," you are doing the same for yourself. Loving you, loving me.

You, too, can learn how to dance through these years. Dance is about learning the next step, opening up, exploring, and moving forward. Come dance with me.

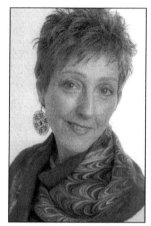

Linda Vettrus-Nichols is an internationally known author and speaker who inspires and teaches talented heart-centered healers and practitioners to face their truth and change what does not serve them. Linda is a Transformational Business Coach and Spiritual thought leader. As a woman filled with LaDestina, a sense of her own destiny, Linda teaches the dance of the Enlightened Woman, the 3 Stages of the Female Psyche, and the Archetype of the Wild Butterfly Woman. She believes in connecting your human experience with your soul and being the shining star you came here to be with all of your flaws, with all of your faults, and with all of your brilliance.

Learn more: www.EvolutionaryHealer.com
Email: linda@evolutionaryhealer.com

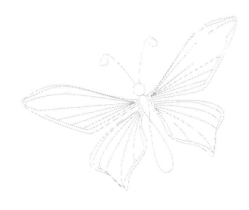

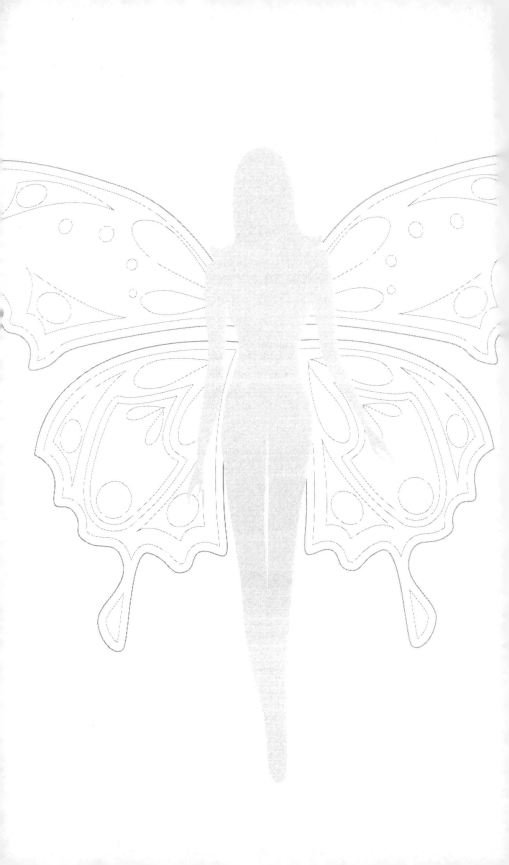

25

Menopause vs. Partial Hysterectomy

LYNNE WADSWORTH

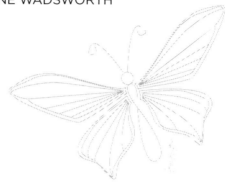

When I had a hysterectomy at age thirty-nine, I thought the silver lining was that I would miss out on menopause. I should be so lucky! Rather than remove my ovaries, my doctor chose to laser off all the endometriosis on my ovaries and "save them." He firmly believed this was the best option for me. However, I was not so happy. I just wanted it all over and done with.

For the next several years, I definitely felt better than I had before my hysterectomy. Then, in my mid to late forties, I began to notice some marked changes in how I felt. I was lethargic and grumpy, had breast tenderness again, had trouble sleeping, and would vacillate between hot and cold. Then came the night sweats. If you've been through them you know how awful they can be—like heat rising from the inside out!

Unaware of healthy, natural alternatives, I went on hormone replacement therapy. I cannot say it helped. It didn't *feel* like it did. I seemed to feel even grumpier, more emotional, and sleep-deprived as the years went on.

I'm a migraine sufferer. I started with migraines after having my first child. In my younger years, the headaches were infrequent and fairly easily treated. However, upon my move to Florida, they intensified with the added components of weather, such as barometric changes, humidity, high heat, blistering sun, thunderstorms, and hurricanes. Then my sinuses and allergies came into play as well. Menopause seemed to intensify my migraines tremendously.

And so began one of the worst periods of my life—dealing with menopause, intensified headaches, and a slew of medications to add to my woes. Of course, I had pain killers and preventatives for my migraines, then followed by medication for stomach and gastric issues brought on as a result of all the migraine medications. I felt like a walking pill bottle. As many women going through "The Change " have experienced, these times can be miserable. But, I discovered, they don't have to be.

After being on hormone replacement therapy for several years, I began to follow Dr. John R. Lee, who became a very well known proponent of "menopause by natural means." I was even lucky enough to hear him live as a speaker before he passed away. His information was scientific, personal, and insightful. Even my gynecologist at the time was following his protocols, and I was glad to have found someone who recommended a more natural approach.

I worked with progesterone cream for quite a while and had some success with it, but after a while, it was not quite so effective. The hot flashes, night sweats, hot and cold feelings, and grumpiness never seemed to fully go away. At that point, all I knew was that I needed help and I did not want to have to go back to using synthetic drugs.

About four years ago, I was introduced to a wonderful naturopath who has helped me in many areas of my overall health. She supports Dr. Lee's alternative methods and uses a holistic approach with her clients. She recommended a product by Dr. Chi called Myomin. Myomin is an estrogen balancing formula and immunity enhancer. It inhibits the aromatase enzyme (balances excess estrogen) and competes with estradiol at the target cell's estrogen receptor. It helps with a wide range of issues, from colon polyps to ovarian, cervical, uterine, and breast cancer.

I have used this product now for quite a few years as I have been going through the tail end of menopause. It has been a tremendous help with my sleep and has helped me feel more stable and balanced. It has even stopped the night sweats.

I have to say that many of my menopausal years were a struggle for me. Even now, from time to time I have issues with symptoms of menopause. I have, however, learned how and when to change my dose of Myomin, and as long as I am consistent with that, I stay well.

As a Board Certified Health Coach who fully believes in natural approaches to health, I wish I had had the resources and knowledge I have now when I began my menopausal phase. Now I know how much certain foods help in stabilizing and balancing the body, which helps tremendously through menopause. I now know that there are options other than traditional hormone replacement therapy.

The worst part of menopause for me has been the increase in migraines. It is ironic, really, because for many women, going through menopause decreases or eliminates migraines completely. Over the past two years, though, I have been able to use a more holistic and natural approach to reducing and helping my migraines. Strange as it sounds, even now, my migraines seem to be cyclic to some degree—some occurring at the same time each month. Luckily, I am now able to perform maintenance/preventative routines to help prevent migraines with the tools of healthy eating, exercise, and the use of specific essential oils. A combination of lavender oil, peppermint oil, and frankincense on the back of my neck and forehead has given me a great deal of relief from headaches.

Balancing hormones and managing harmful metabolites by eating a healthy diet rich in phytoestrogens and other essential nutrients, exercising, and managing weight can help reduce uncomfortable symptoms associated with PMS and the transition through menopause, as well as support healthy bones, heart, breast tissue, and other body structures and functions as a woman ages. In addition, vitamin-type complexes in essential oils can support hormone balance throughout the phases of a woman's life.

Specific essential oils help women manage the symptoms of PMS and the transitional phases of menopause in a natural, effective way.

Menopause can be a time of sleeplessness. There are oils to help with that, as well, including lavender oil for a sense of calm and relaxation and blends that foster a sense of peace and well-being for restful sleep.

No woman really knows what to expect of menopause until she's in it. If, like me, you had a partial hysterectomy, you may think that menopause will either pass you by or will be negligible. For me, that hasn't been the case. Even with a partial hysterectomy, I've experienced symptoms, pain, and changes.

I remember thinking I wasn't so bad—that I wasn't that emotional and cranky with my family—but believe me, they would tell a different story! We don't always see it in ourselves, but our families will often be more than willing to point it out to us. If that's you, it's time to seek help. Natural help! You don't have to suffer through menopause; the symptoms can be managed through natural methods.

Find some friends who can support you and encourage you while you are going through this—but be wary of friends who are negative and will only drag you down. Find a small support group of trusted friends and family who can help you get through menopause in a natural and positive way. A health coach can support and encourage you through this phase of your life and walk you through some of the many ways to manage symptoms.

Getting through to the other side can be life-changing and wonderful. So here's to us—to the challenges and struggles, but especially to life "on the other side!" We can do this, and we can do it gracefully.

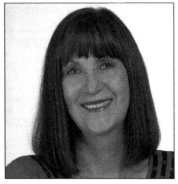

Lynne Wadsworth, a board certified Holistic Health Coach (AADP) and a graduate of the Institute for Integrative Nutrition, creates personalized programs for weight loss, healthy living, balance, and self-esteem. Having suffered from continual, chronic, and debilitating migraines for many years, Lynn specializes in achieving migraine relief through dietary changes, relaxation, and other tested and proven techniques. Learn more at www.holistic-healthandwellness.com or find her on Facebook at www.facebook.com/holistichealthandwellnessllc.

For more information, please visit us at

www.menopausemavens.com